YOUR GUIDE TO BREAST HEALTH

EXPERTS
IN PINK

CINDY PAPALE-HAMMONTREE
SABRINA HERNANDEZ-CANO, RDN, CDE, NC

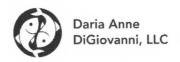

Daria Anne
DiGiovanni, LLC

Copyright© 2018

Cindy Papale-Hammontree

Sabrina Hernandez-Cano

All rights reserved.

ISBN 13: 978-0-692-14673-6

Printed in the United States of America

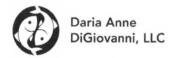

Daria Anne
DiGiovanni, LLC

Experts in Pink

Your Guide to Breast Health

Cindy Papale-Hammontree

Sabrina Hernandez-Cano, RDN, CDE, NC

Contributors

Monica Yepes, M.D.; Alejandro Badia M.D.; Jill Waibel, M.D.; Deirdre Marshall, M.D.; Erin Wolfe, B.S.; Roger Kouri, M.D.; Daniel Calva-Cerqueiral, M.D.; Richard Nadal, M.D.; Beatriz Amendola, M.D.; Carmen Calfa, M.D.; Javier Jimenez, M.D.; Susan Kesmodel, M.D.; Rita Dargham, D.M.D.; Dennis Patin, M.D.; Moises Jacobs, M.D.; Alex Fagenson, M.D.; Mariana Khawand, M.D.; Khin M. Zaw. M.D.; Don Torok, Ph.D., F.A.C.S.M.; Sameet Kumar, Ph.D.; Cristina Pozo-Kaderman, Ph.D; Janet Villalobos, A.R.N.P; Jonathan David, Esq.; Suzanne Moe; Gary Barg, CEO & Editor-in-Chief of Today's Caregiver; Tamera Anderson-Hanna, L.M.C.; Marilyn Van Houten, R.N. M.S., C.C.M; Sam Rivera.

LEGAL DISCLAIMER

Cancer is a serious medical condition. It requires professional medical care. The information in this book is presented as a guide to help you in your journey.

None of the authors, contributors, Daria Anne DiGiovanni LLC, or anyone associated with *Experts in Pink: Your Guide to Breast Health* or the information contained in this book aim to substitute for medical care. Use this book to help you ask questions, discuss, and become proactive together with your choice of medical professional team.

The authors, publisher or anyone associated with the Experts in Pink book, website, or any entity under this name are not responsible or liable for any loss or damage allegedly arising from any information or suggestion in the Experts in Pink book.

Our purpose is to bring light and awareness to the many options available in breast cancer care and to help make the journey one filled with peace, hope, and lots of love and laughter.

REVIEWS

"It's so important to be informed as a woman. Cindy and Sabrina provide a compassionate and detailed look into the impact and most importantly the solutions to empowering yourself when dealing with Breast Cancer. Thank you ladies!"

— Mariel Hemingway

"It's life's biggest challenges that usually lead us to understand our purpose and what we're here for. Cindy Papale Hammontree and Sabrina Hernandez Cano are two amazing women who have turned their challenges, into opportunities to enlighten and teach others. 'Experts In Pink' is a guide that will help educate women on breast cancer health for generations to come. It is an honor to call these two ladies friends."

— Tracy Wilson Mourning, Founder of Honey Shine Mentoring Program and wife of former Miami Heat Player Alonso Mourning.

Reviews

"*Experts in Pink*, is just that, a collection or rather a community, of people who offer their expertise on what happens before and after breast cancer diagnosis. But, this book offers so much more than that. In addition to the invaluable medical and clinical information from some of the most well-respected, renowned physicians in this field, you learn that the journey is long and winding, with several forks in the road. You discover that 'chemo brain' is a real thing and the cardiac effects of chemotherapy are also highlighted. The importance of dental care is discussed, and you are reminded how nutrition and exercise are of paramount importance. You learn the pivotal role spirituality plays and that includes my love, music!! Who knew! And let's not forget the vital role of caregiver, that person in your corner that champions you every step of the way. Consider this book yet another cheerleader, screaming and doing flips from the sidelines, chanting 'You got this', 'You can do it!' Because, of course you can!"

— JULIE GUY, MORNING RADIO HOST, LITE 101.5 FM

"Sabrina and Cindy are enlightening us once again with the ongoing intelligence attached to the continuing battle with breast cancer. Their relentless commitment is a testament to their passion and dedication to this cause."

— MARI SECADA, SECADA PRODUCTIONS, INC.

DEDICATION

It is with pleasure and love as a sister that I dedicate Experts in Pink to my dear brother Mike Papale, who lost his battle to colon cancer in June, 2010 at the young age of 51. Mike was an amazing, loving guy who always went out of his way to help others. We were all devastated to hear the news of his diagnosis, but Mike always remained positive. Rarely did he complain about his pain.

Because he was still a child inside a young man's body, Mike could be immature at times. I remember back to our school years when he and I had gotten pulled out of class at the same time and thought we were getting kicked out of school. I was scared; Mike was happy. Turned out, we'd been expelled from class because they found out we hadn't had our mandatory polio shots. Upon hearing the news, Mike was NO LONGER happy!

For 30 years he worked at Hollywood Memorial Hospital in the Pedi-ICU Unit, where he saved the lives of many babies. Mike was very close to his co-workers, many of whom he took under his wing. People like Jay Hill, whom he always kept laughing and De Ann Laufenberg, whom he loved like a sister (and whose family treated him as one of their own).

To Mike's other friends Bobbie Jones and Eileen Watkins, thank you for taking such good care of him during his final days. To his wife Debbie, know that Mike loved you more than anything in this world. He would also have been proud his two children Debbie and Michael, and all eight of his grandchildren. We all miss and love Mike, and know you are resting in peace – another angel watching over your family and friends.

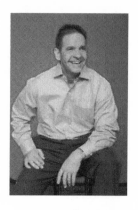

Mike Papale

Much love from your sister,
Cindy Papale-Hammontree

DEDICATION

*In Loving Memory of my Business Partner, Allen Brentenson and my
Brother, Ralph Lazaro Sanchez*

*In loving and unforgettable memory of the best business partner anyone
could ask for. Allen, I know your spirit is still with me and your sky blue
eyes are watching over us all.*
*I feel your pride and your guidance in the raising of "our baby," Humming-
well bar, our humanitarian project of love. Your passion, your words of
encouragement and your business savvy linger. I think about you every
day and I honor every promise I made to you before you left me. Hummingwell's commitment to St. Jude's kids will always be our first priority, while
we continue to wish each and every customer wellness. I love you for all
that you were during your time on earth, and everything you continue to
represent: a good old-fashioned American, a Montana born-and-raised
eagle.*
*Our Humming bird is flying high; you will always be the wind beneath my
wings.*

I love you.
Your "best partner,"
Sabrina

Allen Brentenson graduated from the Thunder-
bird School of Global Management. He was an
International businessman who joined a fortune
500 company and successfully led them through
Latin America and the Caribbean. He served on
the board of directors of Baptist Hospital for
many years and formed the International Divi-
sion at Baptist Health South Florida, where Allen
and Sabrina met and worked together. In 2003,
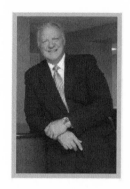
Allen and Sabrina discovered they both shared a
passion for good nutrition and wellness. They founded Scientific Nutrition
and developed Hummingwell wellness bars to bring to the community the
message that delicious food can also be nutritionally sound. After many
trials and the discovery of premium ingredients in Oregon, they took a
chance and developed a bar that has all the goodness of nature with 22 vita-
mins and minerals. Soon after the birth of Hummingwell bars, Allen
received a devastating diagnosis: an uncommon malignant cancer called
angiosarcoma on his forehead. It took his life on January 14, 2015. He leaves
a legacy of leadership and friendship and his partner Sabrina to carry on
the name of their little bird and message of wellness, Hummingwell.

To my brother Ralph Lazaro Sanchez –
a free and kindred spirit whom I lost on
December 26, 2014 from metastatic
prostate cancer – my brother, you abso-
lutely rock! I'm living the life you taught
me to live. Every day is a breath of fresh
ocean air; every minute I hear the sound
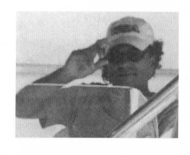
of church bells and know that your spirit is dancing in my heart.

I love and miss you, especially on every Thanksgiving Day to come.
Your sis,
Sabrina

CONTENTS

PREFACE

VINCE PAPALE

When I think of what people say my legacy would be it would be that "he helped someone reach their full potential!" And as you think about it, one of the greatest wastes of all time is the waste of potential and not living life to the fullest. One person I know who is not wasting a second of her life is my beloved and courageous cousin, Cindy Papale-Hammontree.

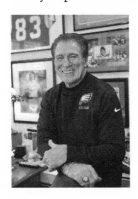

In football, we would not go into a game without a game plan that is well scripted in our playbook. And the same should hold true in life because in this real-world game you'd better be prepared for obstacles and setbacks. In their new book, *Experts In Pink: Your Guide to Breast Health*, Cindy, along with her co-author Sabrina Hernandez-Cano provides you and your caregivers with a winning game plan and strategy to defeat one of the biggest opponents in life...cancer. In this case, breast cancer. Cindy has certainly walked the walk in her 18-year journey as a breast cancer survivor. I believe I have too after kicking colon cancer in the butt for the last 17 years.

One of the keys to survival is atti-tude and, of course, surrounding yourself with a winning team. In trying to come up with something original I keep coming to back to Seal Team Six rowing that boat into the crashing waves and into the sea. Visualize this in the battle vs breast cancer: every person pulling their oar must do it in unison to get through those powerful waves. Each person has to dig deep, ignore the pain, and

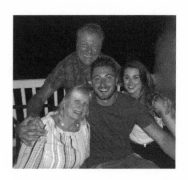

Vince Papale with his wife Janet, daughter Gabriella, and son Vinny

find something inside they never knew existed in order to win that battle. Imagine each oar being stroked by the oncologist, the radiolo-gist, the surgeon, the hospital, the caregiver, the lab tech, the nutri-tionist, and the fitness trainer. The 'cox' is The Family. If one oar is off cadence, the entire boat rocks and swerves out of control, and the whole mission is lost. In Cindy's case, all was in sync, and here she is 18 years later smiling and inspiring. She's helping people reach their full potential by not only surviving but by caregiving, sharing, and inspiring.

I found in my cancer battle that nutrition and fitness were the keys to my survival as well as, of course, attitude and team. Sabrina expands on nutrition in *Experts in Pink* and I'm going to implore you to be in the best physical condition of your lifetime as you head into your Super Bowl game of life.

Cindy is so full of energy and passion that you are going to love her as you read through this book. Yeah, you're gonna laugh and you're gonna cry but more importantly you're going to be inspired and motivated to be the best you can be and not waste your potential. Thanks to research and strong ladies like Cindy and Sabrina it's clear that the impossible is truly possible

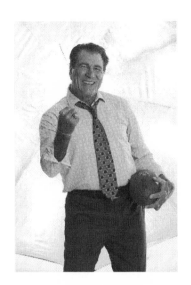

and there will be a cure for cancer. Doing the unthinkable is what defines being Invincible and Cindy, Sabrina and all of us were born to be *Invincible*!

BRCASTRONG

BRCAStrong was founded by Tracy Milgram-Posner in 2015 as a community support group for BRCA positive women and survivors. In 2018 BRCAStrong became a Nonprofit Organization www.brcastrong.org which is built on the very foundation of supporting Previvors and Survivors. Whether routine monitoring or preventative surgery, we can help you through your journey.

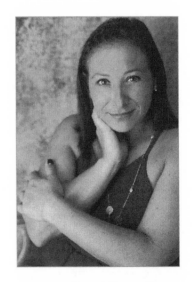

Tracy Milgram-Posner

The diagnosis can be overwhelming and isolating. You are not alone! BRCAStrong will navigate you through the process with others who are making the same decisions and facing the same fears. Empowering women living through their journey and mastectomies is imperative. We can help women network with the right foundation and physicians to properly support their needs. "Our mission is to support, educate, inspire and empower Previvors and Survivors, to eliminate the feeling of isolation." Through the money raised with BRCAStrong funds women in need of bra's or other feminine clothing we will help those women feel whole again. BRCAStrong strives to alleviate the emotional and financial burdens of women facing genetically predisposed breast and/or ovarian cancer through advocacy, direct assistance, empowerment, fundraising initiatives and events.

I underwent genetic testing in my early twenties and learned I was a carrier for the BRCA 2 gene mutation prior to "Angelina Jolie" coming forward to the public with her diagnosis. Prior to her diagnosis there were very limited support groups or even research like there is now. Three months prior to my surgical journey to becoming a Previvor I started BRCAStrong. When I started BRCAStrong my intention was to bring awareness to other women and families, little did I think a couple years later I would have over 2,000 women in a private group posting questions and sharing their stories nationwide.

Becoming a Previvor was not an easy choice, whoever said removing healthy body parts would be easy! "NO ONE EVER." My journey has become my passion and it I will continue to share my experiences with all and make a difference in as many communities as I can. I had participated in a clinical trial (airXpanders), spoke on Capitol Hill in regard to the Patient Education Act, started a Concierge Boutique (UnBRCAble Boutique), Events (Medical Panel & Fashion Shows), Retreat for Survivors and Previvors, Magazine articles, Dateline health and much more.

BRCAStrong is thankful and grateful to have partnered with Cindy Papale-Hammontree and Sabrina Hernandez-Cano. They are both part of our Executive Board Members of BRCAStrong.

Cindy since the first day I met you in person after being social media friends for 2 years I felt your energy was contagious, your story was UnBRCAble and you opened your heart to me that day and felt a connection that would be long lasting. From that day forward in 2018 we have spoken at least twice a day planning what we can do next and how we can get there together. Your team work, dedication and commitment is so admirable.

Sabrina, I heard all about you for months from Cindy and when I met you, I knew why you were her partner in crime. Both of these women in my opinion have such a big heart and great soul. The first time I met Sabrina in person was at the Experts In Pink book signing and she was telling my story. In the middle of Sabrina telling my story she called me up and said this story is s personal lets call Tracy up as tears were running down her face as she greeted me with the tightest hug. From that day forward our bond and relationship has grown.

To Blessed to Be Stressed working with these amazing women and their book that will help millions of women.

For more information visit BCRAstrong.com.

FOREWORD

GAIL IRONSON, PH.D, M.D.

Cindy and Sabrina have teamed up for a third time to make available an outstanding book – a "must-read" for anyone who has or knows anyone with breast cancer, by gathering an incredible group of experts. They have done an amazing job of making their previous books *The Empty Cup Runneth Over and Miami Breast Cancer Experts* even better by updating the contents and adding several chapters to provide readers with the latest treatment options.

The terrific thing about this book is that it covers multiple topics, and does so in a readable, interesting way – enabling us to be better informed about how to cope, what to expect, and how to make wise treatment decisions. It will also help you discuss options with medical personnel.

I first met Cindy over 20 years ago when she was an administrative assistant at the Psychological Services Center at the University of Miami. I was immediately impressed by her bubbly enthusiasm and her ability to make everyone who came to the Psychological Services Center feel comfortable. Her natural inclination to share and help people led to this book (and her previous two) where, in a labor of love, she has transformed her own wrenching experience with breast cancer into a vehicle to educate us about many aspects of dealing with it. She has drawn together an amazing group of experts who write chapters on everything you would ever want to know about this illness. This book takes the mystery and the fear out of breast cancer by making the diagnosis and what happens familiar.

The experts include medical doctors, a nurse, a nutritionist, a mental health professional and a lawyer. In one particularly moving chapter, oncology nurse Janet Villalobos describes the daily ups and downs of treating patients on the front lines (especially children). She also gives some useful advice to cancer patients from years of experience seeing patients go through treatment.

The medical expert coverage of different areas related to breast cancer is extensive. New to this edition is a chapter on imaging and diagnosing BCA. You can tell this chapter is written by an award winning teacher and medical doctor as it gives very clear explanations (including great radiographic pictures) of why the doc might need additional tests for diagnosis and what these tests are. This chapter is particularly helpful because it provides enough information to give the reader an understanding of what to expect during diagnostic procedures, what the doctors look for, and how the diagnosis is made. Thus, you do not feel that you are "in the dark".

Once diagnosed, readers can learn about treatment from the next three chapters. Dr. Susan Kesmodel's brand new chapter on surgery describes the various types of surgeries including lumpectomy and different types of mastectomies. The chapter on Breast Cancer Oncology by Dr. Carmen Calfa describes the various subtypes of cancer, staging, and chemotherapies. It does get technical at times, but remains understandable and transmits much needed information and takes the scariness out of options. Another treatment chapter is the updated chapter by Dr. Beatriz Amendola on Radiation Therapy. She describes advances in radiation therapy including, for example, brachytherapy, in which a radioactive treatment source is placed near or inside the tumor, which spares adjacent tissues from radiation. She makes a comparison to traditional external beam radiation therapy and notes, for example, that brachytherapy drastically reduces the length of treatment. Knowing what to expect during surgery, chemotherapy and radiation that the reader will gain access to in this book can help one be prepared to cope with the treatments.

After surgery, one of the difficult decisions one is faced with is what type of breast reconstruction to have. This book has a set of four chapters that will help guide you. Three of these chapters are new, while the one by Dr. Khouri is updated. Dr. Deirdre Marshall covers the various plastic surgery options, Dr. Khouri discusses autologous breast reconstruction (i.e. using your own tissues and fat grafting). And enhancing the appearance of reconstruction includes two new chapters – one on nipple tattooing (Suzanne Moe) and one on scar rehabilitation (Dr. Jill Waibel).

The next topics provide insight into issues associated with breast cancer treatment and how to deal with it. Some particularly troublesome symptoms include lymphedema, neuropathy and pain: The chapter by Dr. Badia details how to recognize lymphedema, separates fact from fiction, and gives suggestions for ameliorating symptoms. An updated chapter by Dr. Patin offers very useful descriptions and options for treatment for pain. The recognition that breast cancer therapies may have a marked impact on dental health and what to do about it is covered in the new chapter by Dr. Dargham. Finally, potential cardiac complications from specific chemotherapy agents and radiation therapy are part of the thorough picture covered in the new chapter by Dr. Jimenez.

There are several thoughtful chapters on coping with breast cancer and maintaining emotional well-being both for the patient and the caregiver. The signature chapter in this regard is written by an experienced psycho-oncologist, Sameet Kumar, PhD, whom I invite every year to give a lecture in my graduate class of students training to be health psychologists. A new chapter on Yoga and Meditation by Tamara Anderson Hanna explains the many benefits of Yoga and meditation (including a sense of calm) and the importance of finding a practitioner who specializes in Yoga for cancer patients. And this book does not forget about the caregiver : The new chapter by Gary Barg compassionately discusses the challenges involved.

Healthy lifestyles are another major content area with experts' chapters providing up to date information. These will be useful both for people with breast cancer and those who wish to take steps to avoid breast cancer. The updated chapter on nutrition, written by a nutritionist and co-editor of this book, Sabrina Hernandez-Cano, provides expanded information on healthy eating, superfoods, supplements for cancer patients or for prevention, information on weight loss, and wonderful recipes. There is a chapter on obesity from Dr. Moises Jacobs, which has a focus on surgical options. And a most informative chapter on exercise from Don Torok, PhD, gives helpful advice on what general activities to do that actually count as exercise as well as cancer specific suggestions so exercise may be done safely. Exercise is particularly important both for prevention of cancer and enhancing general well-being. In fact, other literature shows that exercising is the equivalent of taking an antidepressant for mild to moderate depression.

Personal stories will help people with cancer to cope with and navigate this difficult illness as well. As Cindy points out, the diagnosis and treatment of breast cancer is undoubtedly difficult and often comes as a shock. Her story beautifully leads you through the adjustments and decisions, and tells you about her exciting journey forward with writing the books to make intricate information reachable. She is a shining example of resilience. Marilyn Van Houten takes us through her inspirational story of the difficulty of finding a lump and getting diagnosed with breast cancer, but also discovers a new world for her and new friends through singing in the "The Heroines Choir."

In addition, this book does not hesitate to discuss difficult issues – it provides information on deeply personal topics such as sex and sexuality from Christina Pozo-Kaderman, Ph.D.. Another difficult concern addressed is what happens if health deteriorates significantly – there is a thorough chapter on palliative care from Dr. Khin M. Zaw and Dr. Mariana Khawand. There is a new chapter by Sam Rivera, who bravely discusses an often forgotten and stigmatized topic – male breast cancer. And finally, there is an informative legal chapter by Jonathan David, esquire.

To conclude, it is estimated that 1 in 8 women will get breast cancer during their lifetimes. The treatment information and decisions one needs to make after being diagnosed with breast cancer can be daunting and overwhelming. This book will undoubtedly help with dealing with and making those decisions. And it will help navigate what comes after the diagnosis. It is a great service that Cindy and Sabrina have done by putting this updated book together and it has my enthusiastic endorsement.

~

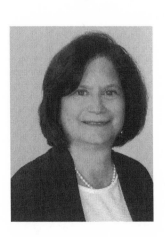

Dr. Gail Ironson is a Professor of Health Psychology and a Board Certified Psychiatrist. She received her Ph.D. from the University of Wisconsin, her M.D. from the University of Miami, and her residency training at Stanford. She has 250 publications in the field of behavioral medicine applied to HIV/AIDS, cancer, and cardiovascular disease, is current President of the Health Division of the International Positive Psychology Association, is past president of the Academy of Behavioral Medicine Research Society

Foreword

(a senior level organization by invitation only), and is a current or past member of the editorial board of five journals (International Journal of Behavioral Medicine, Mind/Body Medicine, AIDS and Behavior, Health Psychology, and Journal of Applied Psychology).

She has directed or co-directed federally funded research studies investigating psychological factors in long survival with HIV/AIDS, stress management in HIV and cancer, massage therapy and immunity, and treatments for recovery from traumatic events. Finally, she set up and runs the trauma treatment program at the University of Miami Psychological Services Center, which makes available to the community (on a sliding scale basis) both traditional (PE, CPT) and newer (EMDR) approaches to treatment. Her current areas of focus include examining positive psychological factors (such as spirituality, compassion, meaning, positive affect, optimism, and emotional expression) and health, and recovery from trauma.

INTRODUCTION

It is with immense pleasure that Sabrina and I welcome you to *Experts in Pink: Your Guide to Breast Health*. In 2014, we set forth to accomplish one simple but important goal with our book *Miami Breast Cancer Experts: Your Indispensable Guide to Breast Health* – to create greater awareness through the eyes of breast cancer survivors and the expertise of medical and healthcare professionals who comprise the wholesale care of a woman's journey through breast cancer diagnosis, treatment, and recovery. Although many books had been published on the topic, never had experts in the field come together to share their knowledge of their specialty. Based on the positive feedback and rave reviews we received, we believe we accomplished our goal.

With *Experts in Pink*, we decided to expand upon the topics to include much-needed information on issues related to breast cancer, including cardiac effects after chemotherapy and radiation therapy by Dr. Javier Jimenez; Yoga and mindfulness by Tamera Anderson; and music therapy and its beneficial effect on the immune system by Marilyn Smith Van Houten. Alejandro Badia, M.D., F.A.C.S., a world-renowned hand and upper extremity surgeon, founder of the Miami-based Badia Hand to Shoulder Center and the innovative creator of OrthoNOW® a unique orthopedic walk-in center national franchise, contributed a comprehensive chapter on lymphedema and neuropathy effects after treatment.

We're confident that you'll find inspiration, education, and hope as you turn the pages of *Experts in Pink* and wish you an abundance of blessings on your journey.

To your health,

Cindy Papale

Author/Survivor/Executive Producer

1

WHERE IT ONCE WAS

CINDY PAPALE-HAMMONTREE

As I sat down to write my third book, *Experts in Pink: Your Guide to Breast Health*, I reflected upon the day I heard those dreaded words, "You have breast cancer," to where I am now. To me, more than anything, cancer was horrifying and dehumanizing. From diagnosis to surgery to treatment to the loss of my breasts, it was a tremendous challenge. It put a strain on my marriage and damaged my relationships with family and friends. Deep in my soul, I thought I was going to die, and I'd never felt so alone.

Eighteen years have since passed from the day of diagnosis with a Stage 1, left breast multifocal (meaning more than one tumor) invasive breast cancer. I no longer feel the desperation and isolation from nearly two decades ago, because I've met the most incredible people. Having breast cancer proved to be a blessing in disguise. Among many fun experiences, I modeled in a breast cancer fashion show with inspiring women in the *Day of Caring* event sponsored by Baptist Hospital in Miami Florida. I'll never forget the exhilaration of walking out on stage in front of 500 people and showing them that I survived.

Flashing back to July 13, 2000, I remember waking up in recovery all alone, listening to all the machines hooked up to me, and being scared. My life as I knew it had dramatically changed. Although I was relieved to learn that the cancer had not spread outside my lymph nodes, knowing it was a multifocal invasive tumor instilled formidable anxiety and concern. My tumor was under 2 centimeters but having three separate ones frightened me. Then, of course, came the nagging question I'm sure most cancer patients ask: "Even though no lymph nodes were involved, did the doctor remove all the cancer?" Yet at the same time, I know excessive worrying about something over which I had no control would only impede my recovery.

Three months later, I had a mammogram on my right breast, which the radiologist said looked suspicious. I elected to have my right breast removed, though it turned out to be benign. Over the following months, I opted to take a drug called Tamoxifen. At that time, the protocol was five years. Chemotherapy was simply too strong for me, so taking Tamoxifen was better than no treatment at all. I did well on the drug; my only symptom was my body temperature fluctuating from hot to cold. Other women I met dealt with much worse symptoms like thinning hair, weight gain, and bone discomfort. I felt terrible for them and thanked God that I didn't have to deal with the same symptoms; I had enough to contend with already, from having no breasts to getting divorced. When I worked up the nerve to date, rarely did I get a second one after going out... and that, my friends, is depressing!

Approximately one year after losing both breasts, I was invited to speak to undergraduate students in a psychology class at the University of Miami, where I shared my breast cancer journey. It was emotional and challenging for me; oftentimes, I'd find myself fighting back tears as I attempted to answer personal questions. However, I knew I had to be honest if I wanted to educate others about the disease.

During that first lecture, it surprised me that many students didn't know much about breast cancer and cancer in general, aside from the fact that there were multiple, distinctive stages and types. Still, I was gratified by their genuine interest in the topic, as evidenced by their sincere attention and variety of questions.

Over the next three years, my speaking engagements throughout Broward and Miami-Dade high schools and colleges led to the publication of my first book, *The Empty Cup Runneth Over*, with my friend and co-author Sabrina Hernandez-Cano. In it, I shared my journey and interviews with several University of Miami cancer specialists who explained in detail important things like mammograms and ultrasounds, how biopsies are performed, and the process of breast reconstruction. I also interviewed six women under the age of 30, who were diagnosed with breast cancer. Each of their inspiring stories became a part of *The Empty Cup Runneth Over*.

The book sold so well at Barnes and Noble and on Amazon over the course of seven years that Sabrina and I decided to write another one. In October 2015, we released *Miami Breast Cancer Experts*. The panel discussion and book signing with physicians at Books and Books in Coral Gables drew a crowd of over 250, and the presentation was live-streamed to over 40,000 people. *Miami Breast Cancer Experts* continues to sell well and garner rave reviews from readers. As of this writing, on October 6, 2018 *Experts in Pink: Your Guide to Breast Health* will be released again at Books and Books in Coral Gables, where physicians will host a panel discussion prior to our book signing.

Breast cancer has taken me on an incredible journey: I've met the most remarkable women and men, appeared on our local Channel 6 station, and had an interview with a wonderful organization called *Living Beyond Breast Cancer* (LBBC), with whom I remain in contact. Currently, I'm collaborating with Peabody Award-winning producer Derek Britt on a feature film and a pilot series inspired by my breast cancer journey.

I truly believe that we live our lives not only for ourselves, but for others who need us to remain strong and push through. It's important to show other breast cancer survivors that they too, can be strong, and that they are not alone. To feel helpless, as if your soul has slipped away, is normal. But for me, the biggest challenge was silencing my mind after my initial diagnosis. Thoughts like, *how will I look with no breasts?* and *am I going to die?* reverberated through my brain. For sure, diagnosis and treatment for breast cancer initiates a unique and individual journey for each patient. I've come to view it as my blessing in disguise and I refuse to be a victim!

I am thrilled for you to discover the most up-to-date information about treatments, contributed by multiple talented and accomplished physicians – all of whom I know personally. Some are even my own doctors. About a year ago, a friend referred me to Dr. Javier Jimenez, a cardiologist at South Miami Hospital, who wrote a chapter in this book on cardiac effects after chemo and radiation therapy. I credit him with preserving my sanity after I had difficulty adjusting to a medication prescribed by another cardiologist for hypertension and cholesterol. Dr. Jimenez offers a unique combination of top-level science and medicine within a supportive atmosphere – truly the best of both dimensions of care.

My experience with breast cancer also connected me with Dr. Carmen Calfa, a breast medical oncologist at the University of Miami Sylvester Comprehensive Care Center. Like Dr. Jimenez, Dr. Calfa demonstrates admirable compassion for all her patients. Her chapter on breast medical oncology provides vital information on the latest level of treatments.

Ultimately, this book is filled with HOPE, as it should be. Hope should never be taken away from anyone diagnosed with breast cancer. As a survivor, I'm a living example that it can be overcome.

In closing, I'd like to share one of my favorite quotes from Albert Schweitzer:

"In everyone's life at some time, our inner fire goes out. It is then burst into flames by an encounter with another human being. We should all be thankful for those people who rekindle the inner spirit."

~

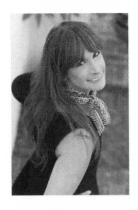

Cindy Papale-Hammontree joined the team at Miami Breast Center in July 2010. A Long Island New York native, she moved to Miami in 1972, where she received a bachelor's degree in Business from the University of Miami. Cindy's boundless passion for helping other breast cancer survivors became even more pronounced in the aftermath of her own diagnosis and treatment in July 2000. She has appeared on the South Florida Today Show and 101.5 LITE FM Radio. Cindy is in the process of collaborating with Peabody Award winning producer Derek Britt on a feature film inspired by her breast cancer journey. Find her on Facebook as Cindy Papale, follow her on Twitter @PapaleCindy, and contact her at the Miami Breast Center.

Miami Breast Cancer Experts: Your Indispensable Guide to Breast Health:
https://www.amazon.com/Miami-Breast-Cancer-Experts-Indispensable/dp/0692499393

Experts In Pink: Your Guide to Breast Health:
https://www.amazon.com/Experts-Pink-Guide-Breast-Health/dp/0692146733

Other ways to connect with me:
http://www.theemptycuprunnethover.com
http://www.facebook.com/cindypapale
http://twitter.com/papalecindy

2

BREAST IMAGING AND BREAST CANCER DIAGNOSIS: WHAT EVERY WOMAN SHOULD KNOW

MONICA YEPES, M.D.

In today's high tech-world the development of multiple innovative technologies for the detection and diagnosis of breast cancer, as well as the wide diffusion of information, may make it difficult to understand what the best process may be for you, as a patient. To help address this question, this chapter will review the current evidence-based recommendations for breast cancer screening and breast cancer diagnosis in patients of average and increased risk for breast cancer. It will also review the different imaging modalities including mammography, ultrasound, MRI, contrast-enhanced mammography, and molecular breast imaging such as Breast Specific Gamma Imaging, analyzing the benefits, limitations, and possible harms of each.

Breast Cancer Screening and Mammography

Breast cancer is the most frequent cancer presenting in women (1) and the second cause of death due to cancer after lung cancer (2). It is estimated that 1 in every 8 women will develop breast cancer in their lifetime, for an average lifetime risk of 12%. In 2018, 2666,120 new cases of invasive cancer are expected in the U.S, with 63,960 new cases of non-invasive (in situ) breast cancer (1).

Mammographic screening for breast cancer is one of the most studied and yet controversial subjects of modern medicine. Since the introduction of dedicated, technically appropriate mammographic screening technology, the natural history of breast cancer changed from the diagnosis of large, palpable tumors, usually 3 centimeters (cm) in size or greater with metastasis to the axillary lymph nodes and survival rates at 5 years of 75.2%, to the diagnosis of smaller non-palpable tumors with an average size of 1.4 cm and negative axillary lymph nodes, translating into 5-year survival rates of 90.6 to 98.6% for these early stage tumors (2).

Controversy

Despite important technological limitations of early mammograms performed from the 1970s to the 1990s, randomized controlled trials (considered the gold standard for research) performed at that time, which compared breast cancer mortality in women who underwent screening mammography to those who did not, proved that there was a 15-17% mortality reduction in women who were "invited" to participate in the trials (even though less than 50% of the women "invited" actually participated in the screening trial in a consistent manner). Subsequent analysis of the patients who *did* participate in the trials demonstrated that the mortality reduction was 24-41% even in the younger, most controversial, 40 to 50 age group (3,4). Unfortunately, we cannot obtain information from randomized controlled trials using the results of modern technology (which might prove a greater survival benefit), as it would be unethical to deny patients mammographic screening based on what we know about the benefit of screening at this time.

Nevertheless, multiple large population-based, observational, nonrandomized trials performed in Europe and Canada have demonstrated an even greater mortality reduction of 30% to 48%, including the 40 to 50-year age group (5,6,7).

So why the controversy?

It revolves around the harms versus benefits of screening mammography. The harms include the anxiety and extra cost produced by the "false positive" diagnosis of mammography when an abnormal finding is seen on a mammogram but is not cancer, the added radiation, the amount and cost of recommended mammograms, and the possibility of over-diagnosing and over-treating breast cancer.

To answer these questions, we must consider the following:

Most women have greater anxiety of presenting with a late-cancer diagnosis than of having to return for additional testing or of undergoing a biopsy. With appropriate communication and information, most women are extremely grateful when they receive a negative result after an abnormal imaging finding. The radiation dose of mammography is extremely small, and the potential risk of causing a fatal breast cancer is far lower than the benefit of diagnosing an early cancer before it becomes palpable (8,9).

The cost of a screening program is offset by reducing the cost of advanced treatment (more extensive surgery, chemotherapy and radiation), as well as minimizing the patients' disability and loss of work-time required for more advanced cancers. While the cost to society of early detection may influence the negative campaign against screening mammography, there is undeniable and incontrovertible evidence that early detection is beneficial to the individual.

And finally, huge strides are being made to correctly identify each patient's own subtype of cancer through genetic profiling to determine the appropriate treatment and minimize the possibility of over-treatment.

Mammographic Screening Recommendations

Based on all these considerations, the American College of Radiology has made the following recommendations (10):

Patients with an average lifetime risk should begin yearly screening at age 40.

Patients who have a first degree relative (mother, sister, father, brother) with breast cancer diagnosed before age 50 should begin screening 10 years prior to the earliest relative's diagnosis. i.e.: if the patient's mother was diagnosed at 45, she should begin at 35.

Special Considerations for High-Risk Patients:

Patients who have been diagnosed with genetic mutations known to cause breast cancer such as BRCA 1 and 2 should begin mammographic screening at no later than 30, and no earlier than 25. Patients with other recently found mutations such as Li-Fraumeni, PTEN, CDHi, PALB 2, CHEK 2, and ATM should also begin early screening based on the age of breast cancer presentation in the family history. Patients who have received high dose chest radiation before the age of 30 should begin mammographic screening 8 years after completion of therapy or at age 25 (whichever comes last) due to the increased risk for radiation induced cancer. These patients should also have yearly screening with breast MRI in addition to mammography (see section on breast MRI) (11, 12).

More recently, due to the elevated risk of breast cancer of early presentation and aggressiveness in the African American population, the American College of Radiology has recommended that these patients undergo risk assessment at the age of 30 to determine whether early screening is warranted (12).

When Should You Stop Screening?

This is an often-asked question: the answer varies from woman to woman. The primary objective of breast cancer screening is to reduce the probability of dying of breast cancer and therefore the following questions should be taken into consideration:

1. Is the patient healthy enough to undergo treatment of breast cancer if diagnosed? If she is too ill because of other disease processes (such as heart disease, severe strokes, kidney failure or other cancers), then she will not benefit from a cancer diagnosis as she will likely not be healthy enough to be treated, and therefore should not be screened.
2. Even if she is healthy, does she wish to undergo further procedures and treatment?

These are things that each patient should discuss with her doctor before screening is performed.

A general rule recommended by the American College of Radiology and the American Cancer Society: women should continue mammographic screening as long as they have a 10-year life expectancy.

Technique

A 2D mammogram consists of 2 views for each breast obtained from different angles to obtain a 3-dimensional evaluation of the breast (craniocaudal and mediolateral oblique views). The breast is compressed between two plates, one of which is a specialized detector. The X-ray penetrates the breast, is absorbed by the detector, and digitally translated into an image. Although very uncomfortable, the compression is necessary for multiple reasons: it inhibits the breast from moving while the image is obtained (if there is motion, the image is blurry, not diagnostic, and must be repeated). It also spreads out the breast to decreases its thickness, allowing for images with better contrast and lower doses of radiation as the amount of radiation is also dependent on the breast thickness.

3D Mammogram (tomosynthesis):

With 3D mammography multiple thin, low-dose images are obtained throughout the entire breast volume. These images are then reconstructed so that 1mm slice images can be evaluated. In addition, these images can be reconstructed into "synthetic" 2D views which do not require any additional radiation. The main benefit of 3D technology is that it minimizes the effect of the superimposition of normal and abnormal tissue which occurs on routine 2D views, the greatest cause of false negative mammograms (missed cancer diagnosis) and one of the most important causes of false positive mammograms (abnormal mammographic result with no cancer). Initial concerns regarding the greater dose of radiation when performing tomosynthesis were caused by initial studies that required performing a "combo" consisting of both 2D and 3D mammography. As each of these has the same radiation dose, this "combo" study was equivalent to twice the dose of a regular mammogram. With the advent of the "synthetic" 2D view, the radiation dose of a 3D study is now the same as that of a 2D study (and half the dose of the "combo").

Multiple studies have shown that 3D mammography increases the diagnosis of breast cancer by 27% to 53% (13-15) and decreases the number of call backs due to tissue superimposition for a win-win situation.

A good screening program is expected to identify 3 to 4 cancers for every 1000 patients that are screened. With the inclusion of 3D mammography, an additional 2 – 3 cancers for every 1000 women screened.

Sensitivity and Specificity

Sensitivity is a measure of the probability that mammography will detect cancer and specificity is the probability that an abnormal finding on mammography will be cancer. The sensitivity and specificity of mammography are determined by the mammographic technique, the density of the breast tissue (see section on breast density), the patient's risk factors, and finally by the experience of the radiologist interpreting the study.

The sensitivity and specificity are highest in patients who have fatty breast tissue and is 86% and 97% respectively and lowest in patients with dense breast tissue with sensitivity ranging from 49% to 64% and specificity 89%(16).

What Do We See on A Mammogram?

A mammogram is used to identify signs of breast cancer such as an irregular mass (with or without calcifications), distortion of the normal architecture of the tissue, changes in the skin and nipple (such as thickening retraction or retraction), or abnormal lymph nodes in the axilla (see image 1). Early signs of breast cancer may be small calcifications or areas of asymmetry (see image 2). It is very important to provide prior mammograms for comparison, as a subtle change from one year to another may be the only sign of malignancy. Patients should not be upset by a request to provide prior studies for comparison as this may also decrease the possibility of being called back for additional imaging.

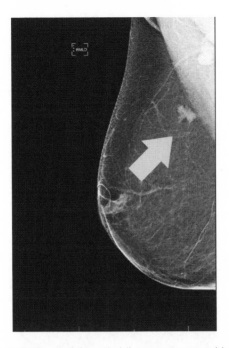

Figure 1: Right mediolateral oblique mammographic view demonstrating a fatty replaced breast with a high density, irregular, spiculated mass with pleomorphic micro calcifications in the posterior aspect of the breast, which is more easily seen in this fatty breast than in a dense breast (compare to figure 3 which is a dense breast).

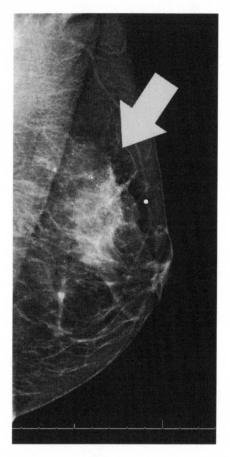

Figure 2: Left Mediolateral oblique mammographic
projection showing cancer presenting as asymmetry with
calcifications (yellow arrow).

Breast Density

A mammogram can also determine the density of the breast tissue.
This refers to the amount of glandular and fibrous tissue compared
to fat in the breast, and is classified into 4 categories based on the
percentage of tissue which is dense:

1. Almost entirely fatty replaced (<25%)
2. Scattered fibroglandular densities (25%-49%)

3. Heterogeneously dense (50-74%)

4. Extremely dense (75% and greater)

The importance of breast density lies in the fact that the dense tissue appears white on a mammogram (as opposed to fat, which appears dark). Breast cancer is also white on a mammogram. Therefore, finding a white cancer on a white mammogram is much more difficult than finding a white cancer in a dark (fatty) breast (see images 1 and 3). Additionally, some studies suggest that the denser tissue may be at higher risk of developing cancer (17). Because of this, some studies recommend that those patients who have increased risk factors for breast cancer and dense breast tissue should have additional screening with breast ultrasound or breast MRI. (see sections on ultrasound and MRI).

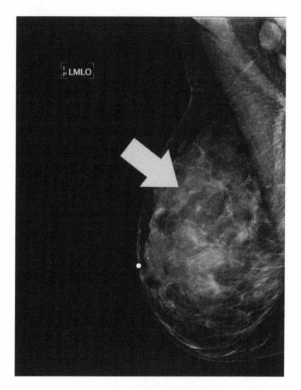

Figure 3: Right Mediolateral oblique mammographic
projection showing a dense (very white) breast, in
which detecting the cancer (yellow arrow) is much
more difficult.

How Do You Obtain and Interpret the Results of Your Mammogram?

A **screening mammogram** is the routine mammogram for patients who have no symptoms and are not being followed for an abnormal finding. The results will be sent to the patient's home within 30 days in the form of a letter which will indicate if the study is normal. If normal, the patient should return in one year; if abnormal, the patient must return for additional imaging. Having to return can be very stressful, yet it is important to understand that the majority of these "call backs" are negative and require no further action. Approximately 10% of these patients will require a biopsy, and of these, only

20-40% may have cancer. Depending upon state legislature, this letter may also inform the patient about her breast density. With this information, and depending upon other risk factors, the patient may elect to have a screening ultrasound or breast MRI (in addition to the mammogram). The referring physician, and the radiologist may assist the patient in making this determination.

A **diagnostic mammogram** is a mammogram performed on patients who have symptoms (such as a lump, changes in the skin, nipple discharge or nipple retraction); or who are "called back" for additional imaging after a screening mammogram; or are being followed every 6 months for what is probably a benign finding. Patients who have a history of breast cancer may also have diagnostic mammograms. These patients will usually be informed of their results at the time of their visit.

The American College of Radiology has standardized the results and recommendations of breast imaging using the BI-RADS (Breast Imaging Reporting and Data System) as follows:

BI-RADS 0: incomplete: additional imaging is necessary, or the patient needs to provide prior studies for comparison before making a definitive recommendation.

BI-RADS 1: negative mammogram, follow up in one year.

BI-RADS 2: benign findings, follow up in one year.

BI-RADS 3: probably benign (less than 2% probability of cancer), recommend a short interval follow up (usually 6 months).

BI-RADS 4: suspicious, needs biopsy.

BI-RADS 5: highly suspicious for malignancy (>95%): needs biopsy.

BI-RADS 6: Biopsy proven cancer (for patients who have already been diagnosed but have not yet completed surgical treatment).

Ultrasound

Ultrasound (US) uses high frequency sound waves (without radiation) to provide additional information which is most useful for evaluating breast masses or areas of asymmetry identified on mammography, and to characterize breast lumps. It can help determine whether a mass is a cyst (made of fluid and usually completely benign) or solid. It will evaluate the shape and margins of solid masses to determine the degree of suspicion for cancer (see image 4). If a mass is seen on ultrasound, it can also be biopsied under ultrasound guidance.

It is also the first study of choice for pregnant patients and patients with symptoms under the age of 30; it may also be considered as first line for patients with certain symptoms between the ages of 30-39.

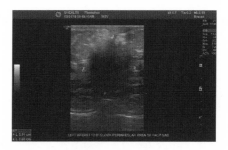

Figure 4. Ultrasound image shows a solid, irregular tumor in the right breast (measured in between calipers) which was not easily visible on mammography in figure 3, as it was obscured by the dense breast tissue.

Screening Ultrasound

Patients with dense breasts, especially those who have additional risk factors, may benefit from additional screening with breast ultrasound (18). Studies have shown that in patients with dense breasts and normal screening mammograms an additional 3-4 cancers for every 1000 screened may be identified. Unfortunately, screening ultrasound comes with a price, as it is also more likely to result in false positive findings and biopsies. It may not be covered by insurance.

Can Ultrasound replace Mammography as the Only Screening Study?

This is an often-asked question. Many women dislike the compression required for mammography as it is uncomfortable and even painful for some. Other women would prefer to avoid the radiation produced by mammography. Unfortunately, ultrasound cannot replace mammography at this time. Mammography is the roadmap that provides the radiologist with the overall view of breast composition and symmetry as well as subtle signs and changes that are not visible on ultrasound such as microcalcifications, areas of asymmetry, or architectural distortion. Ultrasound is a complement to mammography and *never* a replacement.

Tips to reduce the discomfort produced by compression include avoiding scheduling the mammogram during premenstrual and menstrual dates and premedication with low dose ibuprofen.

Contrast Enhanced Spectral Mammography:

This is a mammogram that is obtained after the injection of contrast (iodine). By using a special technique in which 2 images are obtained for each view at different energy levels, subtraction images are created which allow visualization and characterization of masses with high levels of vascularity (similar to MRI). This study only produces 20% more radiation than a regular mammogram and takes approximately 10 minutes to obtain a 2-view study of each breast (4 views total). Studies have shown that in those patients who have suspicious findings on mammography, the sensitivity is 93% vs 78% of non-contrast mammography (19). Additional studies have shown that its diagnostic sensitivity may approach that of MRI (20, 21) in patients with known lesions, and with better specificity (22).

Further evidence is necessary to determine its accuracy as a first line screening modality.

BREAST MRI

Magnetic resonance imaging (MRI) uses the effects of powerful magnetic fields and radiofrequency pulses to cause excitation or resonance of hydrogen atoms that are present in human tissue. This information is then used to create images which can differentiate normal and abnormal breast tissue, fat, water and silicone. By administering contrast (gadolinium), MRI can also detect breast tumors which usually absorb contrast more avidly and quickly than normal breast tissue. By evaluating the tumor's shape and behavior, MRI can offer information regarding whether a tumor is benign or malignant.

Breast MRI is a sensitive imaging modality which has several technical requirements without which it cannot render appropriate information: to date, it must be performed in a closed magnet (open magnets are not appropriate) of at least 1.5 Tesla (this is the measurement of the magnet strength which varies from 1.5 to 3.0 Tesla for clinical purposes), contrast injection is absolutely necessary for tumor evaluation, and the study is highly sensitive to motion: therefore if the patient has moved throughout the study it may need to be repeated. The usual imaging time ranges from 25 to 40 minutes.

Indications for MRI

1. High Risk Screening

As mentioned previously, if a patient is high-risk, defined as greater than 20% lifetime risk of developing breast cancer (11), mammography alone will not suffice for screening. Multiple studies have shown that MRI produces a significant increase in early cancer detection which is not detected on mammography or ultrasound, in the range of 15/1000 with MRI vs 5.4/1000 with mammography and 6/1000 with ultrasound. (23-25).

Patients in this category are those who have genetic mutations such as BRCA 1 and 2, with less frequent mutations such as Li-Fraumeni, Cowden's, and PTEN. More recently, expanded genetic testing has identified other high-risk mutations such as CHEK 2, PALB 2, certain variants of ATM and others (mentioned above). The first-degree family members of women who have been diagnosed with these mutations should be considered high-risk as well until they themselves have been tested.

Some patients have very strong family histories of breast and or ovarian cancer, and yet test negative for genetic mutations. These patients should also be included in the high- risk category, as it is possible they have an unidentified genetic mutation.

Patients who have received radiation to the chest for treatment of mediastinal malignancies such as lymphoma at a young age (between 10 and 30) are also at an increased risk for breast cancer and should be screened with MRI.

Patients with BRCA 1 and 2 mutations should begin screening with mammography and MRI between the ages of 25 and 30 (depending upon the age of presentation of cancer in their family). Patients who have received chest radiation should begin screening 8 years after they completed radiation or at age 25 or whichever comes last. (12)

Patients who have been diagnosed with Lobular Carcinoma In Situ (LCIS), which is a high risk lesion that increases a patient's life-time risk of breast cancer, may also benefit from annual screening with MRI (26).

More recently, the American College of Radiology issued a recommendation for annual screening with MRI for patients who have a personal history of breast cancer, especially those with dense breast tissue or diagnosed by age 50 cancer based on recent evidence that shows a higher incidence of recurrence of breast cancer in these patients than recently expected. (12)

At this time, MRI is not recommended for patients who are at average risk of breast cancer: although MRI is very sensitive for the detection of breast cancer, it is also very sensitive at detecting benign findings which may result in many unnecessary biopsies and follow ups. This must be weighed carefully for patients of average risk. The expense, time and discomfort for the patients are other reasons to not perform this modality routinely.

2. Pre-surgical Evaluation of Breast Cancer

Given the sensitivity of MRI to detect cancers which cannot be seen on mammography and ultrasound, MRI is a valuable tool for detecting additional cancers in patients who have been diagnosed with breast cancer before they are treated. Additional cancers can occur in the same breast in as many as 13-27% (27) of patients (see image 5), and in the contralateral (opposite) breast in as many as 3-5%. (28). It is also helpful to determine the extent of the cancer (which may appear larger than on mammography and ultrasound), as well as to identify whether the nipple or chest wall is compromised (depending upon where the tumor is located). Although MRI is not very specific in evaluating the axillary lymph nodes, it may indicate that they appear abnormal. All this information may be extremely useful to the surgeon and oncologist as it may help determine the extent and type of surgery to be performed (lumpectomy versus mastectomy) or whether the patient may benefit from receiving chemotherapy before going to surgery, also known as neoadjuvant chemotherapy.

Nevertheless, pre-surgical MRI can also lead to more unnecessary biopsies (which can delay the time to surgery), increased anxiety for the patient, and some studies have shown that it may also lead to an increase in the number of mastectomies (29, 30). Therefore, pre-surgical MRI should be recommended on a case-by-case basis. Certain groups of patients have been identified as the most likely to benefit from it: young (pre or peri-menopausal patients), patients with dense breasts in whom mammography is more limited, patients with certain types of cancer which are more likely to present with multiple lesions such as Invasive Lobular Cancer (31), and patients with aggressive cancers such as those that are classified as triple negative (32).

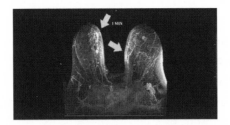

Figure 5 Breast MRI: MIP (Maximum Intensity projection): Showing bilateral breast cancer: yellow arrows denote cancer in each breast. Blue arrow denotes abnormal lymph nodes in the left breast.

3. Occult Breast Primary:

These patients are diagnosed with breast cancer in their lymph nodes, have normal mammograms and ultrasounds. MRI can detect the breast cancer in up to 70% of patients (33, 34).

4. Evaluation of Response to Neoadjuvant Chemotherapy:

Some patients benefit from chemotherapy before surgery because of the size, location or type of breast cancer. MRI has been identified as the best imaging modality to assess whether the tumor is responding to therapy (35) although it may still overestimate or underestimate this response by as much as 29% (36).

5. Problem solving

Occasionally the findings on mammography and ultrasound are equivocal, yet difficult to biopsy. This is especially true in patients with surgical scars (such as a history of lumpectomy and radiation), or other areas of distortion or asymmetry which are difficult to target for biopsy, and in patients with implants that pose a risk for rupture. MRI may be very helpful in ruling out cancer as in these cases the lack of enhancement (absorption of contrast) by the area of concern is highly indicative of a benign process and approaches 100%. This is not true for calcifications, as up to 12% of cancers which present solely as calcifications may be due to cancer, although it will usually be a low grade ductal carcinoma in situ (37, 38).

6. Evaluation of Silicone Implant Integrity

MRI has proven to be highly sensitive and specific for the diagnosis of implant rupture (39, 40). It can detect whether the rupture is contained within the capsule that the body naturally forms around the implant, (named intracapsular rupture), or whether it has breached the capsule (extracapsular rupture). It can also identify whether silicone has leaked to the lymph nodes.

It is important to note that MRI is not necessary for the evaluation of saline implants, as their rupture is usually evident clinically (the breast will feel smaller), or on mammography, where it is seen as a collapsed shell.

Breast Specific Gamma Imaging (BSGI) or Molecular Breast Imaging (MBI)

This is breast imaging performed after the injection of a radiopharmaceutical agent (technetium-99m) with a specialized breast-dedicated camera that can detect the abnormal accumulation of the agent within abnormal breast lesions such as cancer.

Its sensitivity for breast cancer detection is as high as 95%, with good specificity (80%), with some limitations in small (<1 cm) cancers and ductal carcinoma in situ (41). Unlike mammography which only radiates the breast tissue, technetium-99m is distributed throughout the whole body and therefore increases whole body risk, and the risk of radiation induced cancer. Although early results are promising in the diagnostic setting, there are no large trials demonstrating for screening (42).

This study requires compression between 2 plates (slightly less compression than for a mammogram) for each of the four views that are performed for mammography and takes between 45-60 minutes to perform.

Breast Imaging In the Male Patient

Although much less common than in women, breast cancer occurs in 1 of every 1000 men. Approximately 2,550 new cases of invasive breast cancer will occur in men in 2018(1).

Breast cancer in men behaves in a comparable way to breast cancer in women, yet it is more likely to have spread to the axillary lymph nodes at the time of diagnosis.

The most common symptom will be a lump. Any male 25 and over with a palpable lump should begin with a mammogram followed by ultrasound (43). Although the majority of palpable findings in males are due to a benign condition called gynecomastia, which is the development of female-like glandular tissue in the breast, cancer is always a consideration.

Males under the age of 25 should begin the evaluation with ultrasound, followed by mammography only if needed.

Males with breast cancer are at a higher risk of having a genetic mutation such as BRCA1 and 2 and should be tested for mutations. Nevertheless, even those who are found to have a cancer-causing mutation are not recommended to undergo routine screening with mammography, as the most important method for detection is clinical examination.

References

1. National Cancer Institute: Surveillance, Epidemiology and End Results Program: Seer 2018: www. cancer.gov
2. Siegel R, Miller K, Jemal A. Cancer statistics , 2015 . CA Cancer J Clin 2015;65(1):29.
3. Moss SM, Cuckle H, Evans A, Johns L, Waller M, Bobrow

L. Effect of mammographic screening from age 40 years on breast cancer mortality at 10 years' follow-up: a randomised controlled trial. Lancet 2006;368(9552):2053–60.

4. Bjurstam N, Björneld L, Duffy SW, Smith TC, Cahlin E, Eriksson O, et al. The Gothenburg breast screening trial: First results on mortality, incidence, and mode of detection for women ages 39-49 years at randomization. Cancer. 1997;80(11):2091–9.

5. Coldman A, Phillips N, Warren L, Kan L. Breast cancer mortality after screening mammography in British Columbia women. Int J Cancer 2007;120(5):1076–80.

6. Tabar L, Vitak B, Chen TH, Yen AM, Cohen A, Tot T, et al. Swedish two-county trial: impact of mammographic screening on breast cancer mortality during 3 decades - with comments. Radiology 2011;260(3):658–63.

7. Hellquist BN, Czene K, Hj??lm A, Nystr??m L, Jonsson H. Effectiveness of population-based service screening with mammography for women ages 40 to 49 years with a high or low risk of breast cancer: Socioeconomic status, parity, and age at birth of first child. Cancer. 2015;121(2):251–8.

8. Yaffe MJ, Mainprize JG. Risk of radiation-induced breast cancer from mammographic screening. Radiology 2011;258(1):98–105.

9. Miglioretti DL, Lange J, van den Broek JJ, Lee CI, van Ravesteyn NT, Ritley D, et al. Radiation-Induced Breast Cancer Incidence and Mortality From Digital Mammography ScreeningA Modeling StudyRadiation-Induced Breast Cancer From Digital Mammography Screening. Ann Intern Med 2016; 164(4): 205-14.

10. Lee CH, Dershaw DD, Kopans D, Evans P, Monsees B, Monticciolo D, et al. Breast Cancer Screening With Imaging: Recommendations From the Society of Breast Imaging and the ACR on the Use of Mammography,

Breast MRI, Breast Ultrasound, and Other Technologies for the Detection of Clinically Occult Breast Cancer. J Am Coll Radiol [Internet]. Elsevier Inc.; 2010;7(1):18–27.

11. Saslow D, Boetes C, Burke W EA. American Cancer Society guide- lines for breast screening with MRI as an adjunct to mammography. CA Cancer J Clin. 2007;57(57):75–89.

12. Monticciolo, DL, Newell MS, Moy L, Niel B et al. Breast Cancer Screening in Women at Higher-Than-Average Risk: Recommendations From the ACR. JACR 2018.; 15(3): 408-19.

13. Skaane P, Bandos AI, Gullien R, Eben EB, Ekseth U, Haakenaasen U, et al. Comparison of Digital Mammography Alone and Digital Mammography Plus Tomosynthesis in a Population-based Screening Program. Radiology [Internet]. 2013;267(1):47–56.

14. Ciatto S, Houssami N, Bernardi D, Caumo F, Pellegrini M, Brunelli S, et al. Integration of 3D digital mammography with tomosynthesis for population breast-cancer screening (STORM): A prospective comparison study. Lancet Oncol [Internet]. Elsevier Ltd; 2013;14(7):583–9.

15. Skaane P, Bandos A, Eben E, Jebsen in. Two-view digital breast tomosynthesis screening with synthetically reconstructed projection images: comparison with digital breast tomosynthesis with full-field digital. Radiology 2014;271(3):655–63.

16. Kerlikowske K, Carney PA, Geller B et al. Performance of Screening Mammography Among Women with and without a First Degree Relative with Breast Cancer. Ann Intern Med. 2000; 133(11):855-863.

17. Cummings SR, Tice JA, Bauer S, Browner WS et al. Prevention of Breast Cancer in Postmenopausal Women: Approaches to Estimating and Reducing Risk. JNCI

Journal of the National Cancer Institute. 2009; 101(6);384-98.

18. Berg WA, Blume JD, Cormack JB et al. Combined Screening with Ultrasound and Mammography versus Mammography Alone in Women with Elevated Risk of Breast Cancer. JAMA 2008; 299(18): 2151-2163

19. Dromain C, Thibault F, Muller S, Rimareix F, Delaloge S, Tardivon A, et al. Dual-energy contrast-enhanced digital mammography: Initial clinical results. Eur Radiol. 2011;21(3):565–74

20. Francescone MA, Jochelson MS, Dershaw DD, Sung JS, Hughes MC, Zheng J, et al. Low energy mammogram obtained in contrast-enhanced digital mammography (CEDM) is comparable to routine full-field digital mammography (FFDM). Eur J Radiol 2014;83(8):1350–5.

21. Lobbes MBI, Lalji U, Houwers J, Nijssen EC, Nelemans PJ, Van Roozendaal L, et al. Contrast-enhanced spectral mammography in patients referred from the breast cancer screening programme. Eur Radiol. 2014;24(7):1668–76.

22. Fallenberg EM, Dromain C, Diekmann F, Engelken F, Krohn M, Singh JM, et al. Contrast-enhanced spectral mammography versus MRI: Initial results in the detection of breast cancer and assessment of tumour size. Eur Radiol. 2014;24(1):256–64

23. Kriege M, Brekelmans TM, Boetes C, Besnard PE, Zonderland HM, Obdejin IM et al. N Eng J Med. N Engl J Med. 2004;351(5):427–37

24. Kuhl CK, Schrading S, Leutner CC, Morakkabati-Spitz N, Wardelmann E, Fimmers R, et al. Mammography, breast ultrasound, and magnetic resonance imaging for surveillance of women at high familial risk for breast cancer. J Clin Oncol. 2005;23(33):8469–76.

25. Passaperuma K, Warner E, Causer P a, Hill K a, Messner S, Wong JW, et al. Long-term results of screening with

magnetic resonance imaging in women with BRCA mutations. Br J Cancer 2012;107(1):24–30.

26. Bonaccio E, Buys S, Daly MB, Dempsey PJ, Farrar WB, Fleming I, et al. Breast Cancer Screening and Diagnosis. NCCN. 2009;7(10):1060–96.

27. Liberman L, Morris E a, Kim CM, Kaplan JB, Abramson AF, Menell JH, et al. MR Imaging Findings in the Contralateral Breast of Women Breast Cancer. AJR Am J Roentgenol. 2003;(February):333–41

28. Lehman CD, Gastonis C, Kuhl christiane K, Hendrick RE, Ph D, Pisano ED, et al. MRI Evaluation of the Contralateral Breast in Women with Recently Diagnosed Breast Cancer. NEJM 2007;356(13):1295–303

29. Morrow M. Magnetic resonance imaging in breast cancer: One step forward, two steps back? JAMA 2004 Dec 8;292(22):2779–80.

30. Katipamula R, Degnim AC, Hoskin T, Boughey JC, Loprinzi C, Grant CS, et al. Trends in mastectomy rates at the Mayo Clinic Rochester: effect of surgical year and preoperative magnetic resonance imaging. J Clin Oncol 2009;27(25):4082–8.

31. Mann RM, Loo CE, Wobbes T, Bult P, Barentsz JO, Gilhuijs KG a, et al. The impact of preoperative breast MRI on the re-excision rate in invasive lobular carcinoma of the breast. Breast Cancer Res Treat. 2010;119(2):415–22.

32. Bae MS, Moon H-G, Han W, Noh D-Y, Ryu HS, Park I-A, et al. Early Stage Triple-Negative Breast Cancer: Imaging and Clinical-Pathologic Factors Associated with Recurrence. Radiology 2016; 278(2): 356-64.

33. Orel SG, Weinstein SP, Schnall MD, Reynolds C a., Schuchter LM, Fraker DL, et al. Breast MR Imaging in Patients with Axillary Node Metastases and Unknown Primary Malignancy. Radiology. 1999;212(212):543–9.

34. Olson J a, Morris E a, Van Zee KJ, Linehan DC, Borgen PI.

Magnetic resonance imaging facilitates breast conservation for occult breast cancer. Ann Surg Oncol. 2000;7(6):411–5.

35. Hylton NM, Blume JD, Bernreuter WK, Pisano ED, Rosen M a., Morris E a., et al. Locally Advanced Breast Cancer: MR Imaging for Prediction of Response to Neoadjuvant Chemotherapy--Results from ACRIN 6657/I-SPY TRIAL. Radiology. 2012;263(3):663–72.

36. Yeh E, Slanetz P, Kopans DB, Rafferty E, Georgian-smith D, Moy L, et al. MRI in Patients Undergoing Neoadjuvant Chemotherapy for Palpable Breast Cancer. AJR Am J Roentgenol. 2005;(March):868–77.

37. Kuhl CK. BREAST IMAGING: Assessment of BI-RADS Category 4 Lesions with MR Imaging. Radiology. 2015;274(2).

38. Spick C, Szolar DHM, Preidler KW, Tillich M, Reittner P, Baltzer P a. Breast MRI used as a problem-solving tool reliably excludes malignancy. Eur J Radiol 2015;84(1):61–4.

39. Maijers MC, Niessen FB, Veldhuizen JFH, Ritt MJPF, Manoliu R a. MRI screening for silicone breast implant rupture: Accuracy, inter- and intraobserver variability using explantation results as reference standard. Eur Radiol. 2014;24:1167–75.

40. Cher DJ, Conwell J a, Mandel JS. MRI for detecting silicone breast implant rupture: meta-analysis and implications. Ann Plast Surg. 2001;47:367–80.

41. Sun Y, Wei W, Yang HW, Liu JL. Clinical Usefulness of Breast-Specific Gamma Imaging as an Adjunct Modality to Mammography for Diagnosis of Breast Cancer: A Systematic Review and Meta-analysis. European Journal of Nuclear Medicine and Molecular Imaging. 2012;40(3): 450-63.

42. Brem RF, Ruda RC, Yang JL, Rapelyea JA. Breast Specific Imaging for the Detection of Mammographically Occult

Breast Cancer in Women at Increased Risk. Journal of Nuclear Medicine. 2016;57(5):678-84.

43. Mainiero MB, Lourenco AP, Barke LD et al. ACR Appropriate Criteria Evaluation of the Symptomatic Male Breast. JACR 2015; 12(7):678-82.

~

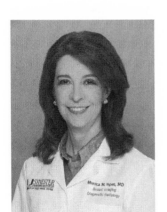

Dr. Monica Yepes is an Associate Professor of Clinical Radiology at the University of Miami, Miller School of Medicine. She is a board-certified radiologist who is fellowship trained in Breast Imaging at the combined Jackson Memorial, University of Miami program. She is originally from Medellin, Colombia where she completed her medical and early radiology training at the Instituto de Ciencias de la Salud, CES.

She has worked at the University of Miami, Miller School of Medicine for the past 17 years, and has served as the Section Chief of Breast Imaging and Director of Breast Imaging services at the Sylvester Comprehensive Cancer Center since 2013. She has also served as fellowship director, director of breast MRI and co-chair of the radiology research committee. She was a member of the American College of Radiology Appropriateness Committee from 2013 to 2017. During this time, she coauthored multiple articles that establish evidence base breast imaging guidelines.

Dr. Yepes has participated and coauthored over 25 peer reviewed articles and 9 book chapters. Due to her dedication to resident teaching, she and earned the Henry H. Lerner Award for teaching excellence in 2008. She is passionate about patient care and minimally invasive techniques for breast biopsy and treatment.

3

ADVANCES IN BREAST CANCER SURGERY: OPTIMIZING OUTCOMES

SUSAN KESMODEL, M.D.

A diagnosis of breast cancer usually elicits a myriad of emotions. Patients are frequently overwhelmed by information regarding the options and recommendations for treatment. There is fear about the side effects from chemotherapy and radiation, the impact of surgery on body image, the potential for cancer to return, and the quality of life after treatment.

Fortunately, our management of breast cancer has changed significantly over the last fifty years, due to numerous studies which have examined alternative treatment options in patients with breast cancer. Advances in systemic therapy (chemotherapy and endocrine therapy) and radiation delivery for breast cancer have allowed for less invasive surgical approaches to be used for patients with equivalent cancer outcomes and improvements in quality of life.

This chapter is an overview of the surgical treatment of breast cancer and outlines the surgical options available to patients with early-stage and advanced disease, newer surgical approaches that are being utilized, how family history and gene mutations affect surgical decisions, and timing of and recovery from surgery. While I have tried to limit the use of medical terms, there are some which are scattered through the text and have been defined. I hope this chapter will help to demystify breast cancer surgery and may be used as a guide for patients with a new diagnosis of breast cancer.

Mastectomy versus Lumpectomy

In the late 19th century, Dr. William Stewart Halsted described a surgical procedure for the management of breast cancer called the radical mastectomy. This was an extensive and disfiguring operation, which removed the breast tissue and overlying skin, the muscles of the chest wall, and the regional lymph nodes. This operation was based on the belief that breast cancer grew in an orderly fashion from the breast to the lymph nodes, and that the likelihood of cancer recurrence would be lower with more extensive surgery. It was also performed at a time when surgery was the only treatment available for patients with breast cancer.

It is now understood that breast cancer is a disease that affects the whole body, and that more extensive surgery does not necessarily improve outcomes. The radical mastectomy has been abandoned in favor of total mastectomy -- a surgery that preserves the muscles of the chest wall and decreases the extent of lymph node removal, after studies demonstrated that radical mastectomy did not improve breast cancer outcomes. As systemic therapies and radiation delivery for breast cancer have improved and as a greater percentage of patients present with early-stage disease due to screening mammography, surgical techniques have also been modified to further decrease the magnitude of surgery and provide better cosmetic results.

There are two primary surgical procedures which may be performed to remove a breast cancer -- mastectomy and lumpectomy. A mastectomy is a procedure which removes the entire breast, and a lumpectomy is a procedure which removes the breast cancer with a margin of normal breast tissue but preserves the majority of the breast. Many patients diagnosed with breast cancer initially want to undergo mastectomy because they think that this will improve long-

34

term survival. However, in patients with early-stage breast cancer, typically defined as those patients with tumors ≤ 5 cm in size, with or without early lymph node involvement, the long-term survival is essentially the same whether a mastectomy or lumpectomy is performed. In the case of lumpectomy, radiation therapy is usually recommended after surgery in order to decrease the risk of local recurrence in the breast. Use of radiation after a lumpectomy also eventually translates into a long-term survival benefit compared to patients undergoing lumpectomy treated without radiation therapy.

There are multiple studies which have compared these two surgical approaches for the management of early-stage breast cancer. All of these studies demonstrate similar survival with the two surgical approaches, with a slightly higher risk of local recurrence in the breast in those patients undergoing lumpectomy. The risk of local recurrence, however, is also dependent on the breast cancer subtype. Those patients with more favorable tumors that are small have a very low risk of tumor recurrence in the breast at 10 years, <10% with the use of appropriate systemic and radiation therapy. For patients with more aggressive breast cancer subtypes, the risk of in-breast tumor recurrence or chest wall recurrence is higher whether a patient has a mastectomy or lumpectomy.

In appropriately selected patients, breast conservation surgery (lumpectomy) allows for preservation of the breast and maintains sensation. However, when considering breast conservation surgery, one needs to balance the oncologic outcome with aesthetic results. Not all patients with early-stage breast cancer are good candidates for lumpectomy. It is important to consider the size of the tumor in rela-tion to the size of the patient's breasts and whether removal of that tumor will result in a favorable appearance. In addition, lumpectomy is usually not considered in patients who cannot receive postopera-tive radiation therapy, unless they are older and have small, favorable tumor types, or in patients where cancer is present in more than one quadrant in the breast.

For those patients who are not good candidates for lumpectomy at diagnosis, there is the option to proceed with a mastectomy with or without reconstruction. An alternative approach is to proceed with upfront systemic therapy, either chemotherapy or endocrine therapy, to try to reduce the size of the tumor and improve the likelihood of successful breast conservation. Overall, the significant improvements in systemic therapy and radiation therapy, and a better understanding of breast cancer tumor biology, have allowed for a decrease in the extent of surgery for breast cancer.

Types of Mastectomy

A mastectomy is a surgical procedure which removes the entire breast. This is a surgical option for patients with early-stage and advanced breast cancer, and may be performed in conjunction with a breast reconstruction procedure. The choice of mastectomy depends on the stage of disease, the potential need for radiation therapy after surgery, and patient preference. The refinement of plastic surgery reconstructive options has resulted in the introduction of more aesthetic mastectomy approaches. As always, the goal is to optimize oncologic outcomes while trying to provide excellent cosmetic results.

Total Mastectomy

Total mastectomy is a procedure that removes the entire breast, including the nipple-areolar complex and, generally, the skin overlying the cancer in the breast. Unlike with a radical mastectomy, the muscles of the chest wall are preserved. This procedure is usually performed when patients are not having breast reconstruction. It may also be recommended for patients with more advanced breast cancers and when it is known that postoperative radiation therapy will be utilized as part of treatment. Patients who undergo a total mastectomy may be candidates for delayed reconstruction either using their own tissue or with breast implants. Total mastectomy may be combined with removal of the axillary lymph nodes, which is known as a *Modified Radical Mastectomy.*

Skin-Sparing Mastectomy

Skin-sparing mastectomy is a newer technique that allows for preservation of the majority of the skin overlying the breast with removal of the nipple-areolar complex. This operation facilitates immediate breast reconstruction and significantly improves the aesthetic outcomes that can be achieved from mastectomy. The surgery is performed through a small circular or elliptical incision in the central breast, which removes the nipple-areolar complex and allows for visualization and removal of the breast tissue. The incision may be extended laterally to obtain additional exposure for removal of the breast tissue if necessary, and sometimes the skin from a biopsy site or overlying a superficial tumor may be included. Skin-sparing mastectomy was initially introduced as an operation for patients with early-stage breast cancer undergoing mastectomy, and in these cases, the oncologic outcomes are comparable to patients treated with total mastectomy. This operation has been extended to patients with more advanced disease, particularly after preoperative chemotherapy.

Nipple-Sparing Mastectomy

Nipple-sparing mastectomy, also referred to as total skin-sparing mastectomy, is a surgical technique that removes the breast tissue, but preserves the entire skin envelope of the breast, including the nipple-areolar complex. This operation was initially developed and utilized for patients undergoing prophylactic mastectomy (a mastectomy when no cancer is present) for risk reduction due to a strong family history of breast cancer or a genetic predisposition for the development of breast cancer, and was subsequently applied to patients with early-stage breast cancer. Initial selection criteria for patients with early-stage breast cancer included tumors that were only in one location in the breast, <2-3 cm in size, at least 2 cm from the nipple-areolar complex, and with no evidence of involvement of the nipple-areolar complex or skin on clinical exam or by imaging. Currently patient selection for this operation have been expanded at many centers and may include patients with more central tumors, multifocal/multicentric tumors (tumors in more than one location in the breast), or more advanced disease, particularly those who respond well to preoperative chemotherapy, as long as there is no direct involvement of the nipple-areolar complex or skin. A variety of incisions may be utilized for this operation including incisions along the inferior aspect of the breast and the side of the breast. Careful surgical planning and meticulous surgical technique to preserve the blood supply to the skin are key to the success of this operation. Problems with healing of the skin of the breast or the nipple-areolar complex may be observed in up to 10% of patients, but skin loss that requires surgical removal of tissue is less common. This mastectomy approach is best suited to patients with small to medium sized breasts without significant sagging of the breasts, but in select cases may be utilized in women with larger breasts. The oncologic safety of nipple-sparing mastectomy is still being evaluated; however, there are several large reports that do not show a significant increase in local regional recurrence rates in patients undergoing this procedure.

Contralateral Prophylactic Mastectomy

Contralateral prophylactic mastectomy (CPM) is a surgical procedure where a healthy, unaffected breast is removed in a patient undergoing surgery for a unilateral breast cancer in the other breast. The rate of CPM has significantly increased in the last 20 years, and some reports estimate that up to 20-25% of women with newly diagnosed breast cancer are undergoing this procedure. There are a wide variety of reasons for this increase, including the use of genetic testing and advances in breast reconstruction techniques. Some of the most commonly identified concerns from patients are the fear of developing a breast cancer in the other breast, although this is generally overestimated, the emotional and quality of life impact of this uncertainty, and the desire for breast symmetry.

Estimating the risk of developing a breast cancer in the other breast is complex, however, some factors that have been shown to increase risk include gene mutations, family history of breast cancer in a first-degree relative, and younger age at diagnosis. While it is known that removing the healthy breast in a patient with a unilateral breast cancer will reduce the risk of cancer in that breast by approximately 90-95%, the impact of this surgery on survival in a patient with breast cancer is less clear. It is also important for patients to know that performing surgery on the other breast has risks due to the increased operative time and complication rates. Therefore, the risks and benefits of the procedure, particularly in terms of complications and the potential impact on long-term outcomes, must be factored into the decision-making.

Axillary Lymph Node Management

Management of the axillary lymph nodes in patients with breast cancer has also evolved. Until twenty-five years ago, when patients were diagnosed with breast cancer, an axillary lymph node dissection (removal of lymph nodes under the arm) would be performed in conjunction with breast surgery to remove the primary tumor. This procedure was performed to obtain information about tumor spread to the lymph nodes, which would help guide physicians in recommendations for additional systemic and radiation therapy, and would also provide local regional disease control. However, as with breast surgery, management of the axilla has improved and the extent of axillary surgery in the majority of patients with breast cancer has been reduced.

Sentinel Lymph Node Dissection

Sentinel lymph node dissection is an operative procedure that is used for the evaluation of regional lymph nodes in patients with cancer. This staging technique was initially developed for and gained widespread clinical acceptance in patients with melanoma. However, in the early 1990's, the value of this procedure for patients with early-stage breast cancer was recognized, and the technique was rapidly applied to these patients as well. Since that time, multiple studies have shown that sentinel lymph node dissection accurately assesses the status of the axillary lymph nodes in patients with early-stage breast cancer without compromising oncologic outcomes. More recent studies have also evaluated the utility and accuracy of this procedure in patients with more advanced breast cancer.

Sentinel lymph node dissection is a targeted sampling of the regional lymph nodes. In patients with breast cancer, it is typically used for assessment of the axillary lymph nodes. The procedure is performed by injecting mapping agents into the breast, which then travel through the breast lymphatics to the lymph nodes. The procedure can be performed with the use of a radioactive tracer and/or a blue dye tracer, and these mapping agents can be injected in multiple locations in the breast preoperatively, such as around the tumor or around the nipple-areolar complex. At the time of surgery, the lymph nodes under the arm that have taken up the mapping agents can be identified and removed for evaluation for the presence of tumor. Further surgery for removal of additional axillary lymph nodes depends on whether the lymph nodes are involved, the number of lymph nodes with cancer, and plans for additional treatment.

Sentinel lymph node dissection has significantly reduced the complications associated with axillary lymph node evaluation in patients with breast cancer. In particular, a substantial reduction in lymphedema (arm swelling) rates has been observed, which translates to improvements in quality of life. More recently, there has been an effort to reduce the extent of axillary surgery even further, by eliminating axillary lymph node evaluation all together in select women with early-stage, favorable breast cancers. This approach must be carefully considered in the context of the multidisciplinary care of the patient and should take into account the patient's health and how the results of axillary lymph node evaluation may change treatment recommendations.

Axillary Lymph Node Dissection

Axillary lymph node dissection is an operation that removes the lymph nodes under the arm. This is a surgery that was utilized for the majority of the 20th century in patients with breast cancer and is still recommended for patients with more advanced disease. The operation may be performed in conjunction with a mastectomy or lumpectomy. When performed with a mastectomy, the lymph node dissection may be done through the same surgical incision as the mastectomy or a separate incision under the arm may be used.

Axillary lymph node dissection provides excellent regional control of breast cancer. However, significant complications may be associated with the procedure including arm swelling, loss of sensation, and a decrease in arm and shoulder mobility. Lymphedema rates generally range from 15-25% and require life-long management.

Oncoplastic Breast Surgery

While lumpectomy is an excellent option for most women with early-stage breast cancer, preservation of the breast is more challenging in some patients. Breast conservation may be problematic in women with multifocal tumors, larger areas of cancer, or poorly located tumors. In patients where >20% of the breast tissue will be removed, the resulting cosmetic outcomes can be quite poor, and the deformity may be further exacerbated by postoperative radiation.

Oncoplastic breast surgery is a technique that involves reshaping of the breast after large volume oncologic resection. This allows for breast conserving surgery in patients who might not be considered good candidates for this approach due to concerns for poor aesthetic outcomes. Although local flaps and implants may be required in some cases, many of the procedures involve volume displacement, where the tissue remaining in the breast after cancer resection is utilized to reshape the breast.

Some oncoplastic breast surgery techniques are simple and do not require any skin resection or a breast lift. These level 1 techniques involve local tissue rearrangements and can be utilized when <20% of the breast tissue is removed. These procedures are generally performed by the breast surgeon alone.

When more complex tissue rearrangements are required and include skin resection or breast lifts, the breast surgeon and plastic surgeon work together to select skin incisions and reconstructive techniques that will allow for appropriate resection of the tumor with preservation of the viability of the remaining breast tissue, skin, and nipple-areolar complex. These are considered level 2 techniques due to the increased complexity. Multiple procedures have been developed for reshaping of the breast, which depend on the size and location of the tumor, the size of the patient's breasts, and the degree of breast sagging. Usually a procedure is also performed on the opposite, unaffected breast for symmetry.

There are several potential advantages to oncoplastic breast surgery when compared to standard lumpectomy. These include a lower rate of positive margins, as a larger volume of tissue may be removed, and the potential to decrease postoperative fluid collections at the lumpectomy site. Superior aesthetic results may be achieved with the combination of oncologic resection and plastic reconstruction that may enhance the appearance of the breast. In addition, reshaping of the breast may make it easier to deliver postoperative radiation therapy.

The oncologic outcomes observed with this approach are comparable to those achieved with lumpectomy or mastectomy. Patient selection for these procedures is key because complication rates may be increased in patients where blood supply to the breast tissue and skin is compromised, such as smokers or diabetics. In addition, in patients with fatty breasts, the fat may not heal as well with tissue rearrangements; therefore, these large volume tissue rearrangements are better suited to patients with denser, glandular breast tissue.

Patients with Genetic Predisposition

A significant increase in knowledge and understanding of genetic predisposition and the development of cancer has occurred over the last twenty years. It is now possible to test for a multitude of genes that are involved in cancer development. Management of these gene mutations depends on numerous factors including the specific mutation, the likelihood of developing cancer, family history, patient age, presence of malignancy, and patient preferences. Approximately 5-10% of breast cancers are associated with gene mutations, with the *BRCA1* and *BRCA2* gene mutations accounting for the majority of these. Review of family history in these patients usually shows multiple first and second-degree relatives with breast or ovarian cancer, frequently with early age onset. Although there has been substantial emphasis on decreasing the extent of surgery in patients with breast cancer and trying to reduce the rate of contralateral prophylactic mastectomy (removal of a breast without cancer), in patients with genetic predisposition syndromes more aggressive surgery is often considered. There are two groups of patients to consider, those patients with a known gene mutation who do not have breast cancer and those patients who have been diagnosed with breast cancer.

Patients without Breast Cancer

Patients with a known genetic predisposition syndrome for breast cancer should undergo a multidisciplinary high-risk evaluation. Since genetic predisposition for breast cancer is often associated with ovarian cancer susceptibility, this evaluation usually includes a breast surgeon, medical oncologist, plastic surgeon, gynecologic oncologist, and a genetic counselor. For certain high-risk syndromes that are associated with gastrointestinal malignancies, this may also include a gastroenterologist. In addition to enhanced surveillance with breast magnetic resonance imaging (MRI) and mammogram starting at an earlier age, these patients may be considered for chemoprevention (risk reducing medications) and may also be candidates for risk-reducing surgery.

Risk-reducing surgery involves surgical removal of an organ at risk before cancer develops. For breast cancer risk-reduction, a bilateral mastectomy may be performed. This surgery has been shown to reduce risk of developing breast cancer by 90-95%. There are currently four high-risk gene mutations for which risk-reducing mastectomy is generally considered, *BRCA1, BRCA2, TP53,* and *PTEN.*

For other gene mutations such as *PALB2* and *CHEK2*, the decision to proceed with risk-reducing surgery is significantly influenced by family history. Prior to risk-reducing surgery, these patients should undergo imaging with breast MRI and mammogram to exclude the presence of malignancy. Depending on the age of the patient, risk-reducing salpingo-oophorectomy (removal of the ovaries and fallopian tubes) may be recommended first. This surgery may reduce the likelihood of developing breast cancer with certain gene mutations, and clearly reduces the risk of developing ovarian or fallopian tube cancer and the mortality associated with these cancers.

Patients undergoing risk-reducing mastectomy are usually considered for skin-sparing or nipple-sparing mastectomy and the procedure is performed in conjunction with a reconstructive surgery. This may be an implant-based reconstruction or tissue reconstruction depending on patient preference and body size.

Patients with Breast Cancer

As the ability to test for gene mutations has increased, many more patients with newly diagnosed breast cancer who also harbor gene mutations are being identified. There are guidelines for testing newly diagnosed patients with breast cancer, and these include young age, strong family history of breast or ovarian cancer or other malignancies, and certain breast cancer subtypes. Decisions regarding surgical management in these patients must take into account the type of gene mutation, age of the patient, stage of the breast cancer, family history, and patient preference.

While patients with gene mutations are candidates for lumpectomy and unilateral mastectomy, just like other patients with breast cancer, with certain gene mutations we know that the risk of developing a cancer in the opposite breast is quite high. This is especially true for patients with *BRCA1* and *BRCA2* mutations, where the risk of developing a breast cancer in the other breast at twenty-five years may be greater than 50%, depending on the age of onset of the first breast cancer. This risk of breast cancer in the other breast is particularly high for patients who are diagnosed with their first breast cancer under the age of 40. For patients who are diagnosed at a later age, the risk is significantly lower. There is also concern about the risk of tumor recurrence or the development of new breast cancers in the affected breast. While removing the other breast reduces the likelihood of developing a cancer in that breast, it is still unknown whether this additional surgery improves long-term outcomes. The decision to do more extensive surgery must also take into account the stage of disease. In patients with advanced breast cancer, the risk of disease recurrence may outweigh the benefit derived from the additional surgery. These are complex decisions that must be individualized for each patient.

Timing of Treatment

The model for the treatment of breast cancer has changed considerably in the past twenty years. Previously, patients with operable breast cancer at diagnosis would have surgery first and then proceed with other types of treatment such as chemotherapy and/or endocrine therapy (systemic therapy) and radiation. Upfront treatment with systemic therapy prior to surgery was usually reserved for patients with advanced breast cancer or those patients who had inoperable disease. Although chemotherapy is still recommended prior to surgery for most patients with advanced breast cancer, it is also now administered prior to surgery in many patients with earlier stage disease.

There are several potential benefits to giving systemic treatment prior to surgery. First, response of the tumor to treatment may be observed, and this can provide information on long-term outcomes. Patients who respond well to systemic therapy prior to surgery usually have better outcomes. This also allows physicians to consider additional systemic treatment after surgery, especially in those patients who do not respond well. Second, the extent of surgery that is required may be reduced. More patients are candidates for breast conservation (lumpectomy) if they receive treatment before surgery, and the number of axillary lymph nodes which must be removed may also be decreased. This usually translates into fewer complications from surgery, faster recovery, and better quality of life. Finally, in patients undergoing mastectomy, more cosmetically favorable mastectomies may be possible which can be combined with breast reconstruction.

There are several different subtypes of breast cancer, and they respond to treatment differently. For some of the more aggressive and faster growing types of breast cancer, treatment with chemotherapy before surgery is very effective. Up to 50% of these patients will have no residual tumor identified at the time of surgery. This has resulted in new studies which are evaluating whether some of these patients can be spared surgery altogether. Currently, surgery is recommended in all patients; however, significantly smaller procedures or more aesthetically favorable surgeries are usually possible.

What to Expect from Surgery

Duration and recovery times for breast cancer surgery are quite variable depending on the surgical procedure utilized.

Lumpectomy

A lumpectomy is usually an outpatient surgical procedure which lasts approximately 1-1.5 hours, depending on the size and location of the tumor, and whether lymph nodes are removed. Prior to surgery, if the tumor in the breast cannot be felt, a marker is placed in the breast so that the site of the tumor may be identified at the time of surgery. If lymph nodes will be removed, mapping agents are injected into the breast before surgery to target removal of axillary lymph nodes. The procedure may be performed with general anesthesia, regional anesthesia (nerve blocks) and sedation, or with local anesthesia and sedation, and is usually based on surgeon and patient preference.

Recovery time from a lumpectomy is about 1-2 weeks. Most patients will resume the majority of their normal activities within 1 week. Patients will be up and walking around the same day as the surgery and are encouraged to walk daily after the surgery. Light lifting and movement of the arm on the side of the surgery is allowed and recommended. More strenuous physical activity is usually restricted for the first 2-4 weeks. If lymph nodes are removed at the time of surgery, stretching exercises to increase movement of the shoulder and arm on the side of the surgery are started 1-2 weeks after the procedure. Absorbable sutures (stitches) which are below the skin and do not need to be removed and surgical glue are used to close the incisions and no local wound care is needed.

Mastectomy without Reconstruction

Mastectomy without reconstruction is a fairly common procedure which is performed for patients with breast cancer. This procedure requires 1.5-2 hours to complete and is slightly longer when axillary lymph nodes are removed. The procedure is regularly performed with general anesthesia but can also be done with regional blocks and sedation. This may be an outpatient procedure, but most patients will remain in the hospital for 1 night after surgery.

Patients who undergo mastectomy will have 1-2 drains placed at the time of surgery to prevent fluid from accumulating at the site of surgery. These drains are emptied twice a day and the volume is recorded. The drains are removed in the clinic 1-3 weeks after the surgery, once the output has decreased. Patients should be walking around the day after surgery, and the majority of patients will resume most of their normal activities within 4 weeks. More strenuous physical activity is usually restricted for the first 2-4 weeks after surgery. Patients undergoing mastectomy, particularly those who have axillary lymph nodes removed, may have more trouble regaining full-range of motion of the shoulder and arm on the side of the surgery. If patients are unable to achieve full-range of motion with home stretching exercises, a formal physical therapy regimen may be required. Absorbable sutures which are below the skin and do not need to be removed and surgical glue are used to close the incisions and no local wound care is needed.

Mastectomy with Reconstruction

Recovery from a mastectomy with reconstruction mainly depends on the type of reconstructive procedure performed. These surgeries are usually 3-4 hours in duration when implant-based reconstruction is done, but can be much longer when complex tissue reconstruction is performed. The advantages and disadvantages of the various reconstructive procedures are extensively reviewed with patients before surgery so that there is an understanding of the magnitude of the procedure and the recovery time.

When implant-based reconstruction is used, patients usually stay in the hospital for 1 night and recovery time is similar to that for a mastectomy without reconstruction. Drains are placed at the time of surgery and these are removed in the clinic 2-4 weeks after surgery. Most patients will be out of bed and walking around one day after the surgery. Light activity with the arm on the side of the surgery is permitted immediately after the surgery, as well as light stretching exercises. More vigorous activity and stretching of the arm and shoulder are usually limited for the 2-4 weeks.

Tissue-based reconstructions, where the tissue typically comes from the abdominal wall and back, are more complex and patients may stay in the hospital for 3-7 days. This is usually to provide adequate pain control, to monitor the viability of the reconstruction, and to observe for postoperative complications. Similar to implant-based reconstruction, patients will have drains which need to be emptied. The recovery time from tissue-based reconstructions is longer and may take several months before patients resume their normal activities and exercise routines.

Conclusion

The surgical management of breast cancer has changed dramatically, evolving from extensive operations with significant disfigurement to procedures which provide both optimal oncologic outcomes and excellent aesthetic results. As new treatments for breast cancer become available, surgical techniques and interventions for breast cancer will continue to be refined and individualized for each patient.

Dr. Susan Kesmodel is a surgical oncologist and Board-Certified Surgeon who specializes in the treatment of benign and malignant breast diseases and high-risk skin malignancies including melanoma. She has expertise in skin-sparing and nipple-sparing mastectomy, prophylactic breast surgery for high-risk patients, and sentinel lymph node biopsy and lymphadenectomy for patients with breast and skin cancer. Her research interests include optimizing local regional therapy for patients with breast cancer and the use of neoadjuvant endocrine therapy.

References

1. Fisher B, Anderson S, Bryant J, Margolese RG, Deutsch M, Fisher ER, Jeong JH, Wolmark N. Twenty-year follow-up of a randomized trial comparing total mastectomy, lumpectomy, and lumpectomy plus irradiation for the treatment of invasive breast cancer. N Engl J Med. 2002 Oct 17;347(16):1233-41.

2. Wang F, Peled AW, Garwood E, Fiscalini AS, Sbitany H, Foster RD, Alvarado M, Ewing C, Hwang ES, Esserman LJ. Total skin-sparing mastectomy and immediate breast reconstruction: an evolution of technique and assessment of outcomes. Ann Surg Oncol. 2014 Oct;21(10):3223-30.

3. Smith BL, Tang R, Rai U, Plichta JK, Colwell AS, Gadd MA, Specht MC, Austen WG Jr, Coopey SB. Oncologic Safety of Nipple-Sparing Mastectomy in Women with Breast Cancer. J Am Coll Surg. 2017 Sep;225(3):361-365.

4. Krag DN, Anderson SJ, Julian TB, Brown AM, Harlow SP, Costantino JP, Ashikaga T, Weaver DL, Mamounas EP, Jalovec LM, Frazier TG, Noyes RD, Robidoux A, Scarth HM, Wolmark N. Sentinel-lymph-node resection compared with conventional axillary-lymph-node

dissection in clinically node-negative patients with breast cancer: overall survival findings from the NSABP B-32 randomised phase 3 trial. Lancet Oncol. 2010 Oct;11(10):927-33.

5. Giuliano AE, Ballman KV, McCall L, Beitsch PD, Brennan MB, Kelemen PR, Ollila DW, Hansen NM, Whitworth PW, Blumencranz PW, Leitch AM, Saha S, Hunt KK, Morrow M. Effect of Axillary Dissection vs No Axillary Dissection on 10-Year Overall Survival Among Women With Invasive Breast Cancer and Sentinel Node Metastasis: The ACOSOG Z0011 (Alliance) Randomized Clinical Trial. JAMA. 2017 Sep 12;318(10):918-926.

6. Clough KB, Benyahi D, Nos C, Charles C, Sarfati I. Oncoplastic surgery: pushing the limits of breast-conserving surgery. Breast J. 2015 Mar-Apr;21(2):140-6.

7. Green L, Meric-Bernstam F. Risk of Ipsilateral and Contralateral Cancer in BRCA Mutation Carriers with Breast Cancer. Curr Breast Cancer Rep. 2011 Sep 1;3(3):151-155.

8. Graeser MK, Engel C, Rhiem K, Gadzicki D, Bick U, Kast K, Froster UG, Schlehe B, Bechtold A, Arnold N, Preisler-Adams S, Nestle-Kraemling C, Zaino M, Loeffler M, Kiechle M, Meindl A, Varga D, Schmutzler RK. Contralateral breast cancer risk in BRCA1 and BRCA2 mutation carriers. J Clin Oncol. 2009 Dec 10;27(35):5887-92.

9. Steenbruggen TG, van Ramshorst MS, Kok M, Linn SC, Smorenburg CH, Sonke GS. Neoadjuvant Therapy for Breast Cancer: Established Concepts and Emerging Strategies. Drugs. 2017 Aug;77(12):1313-1336.

10. Handbook of Breast Cancer and Related Breast Disease. Tkaczuk KHR, Kesmodel SB, Feigenberg SJ, eds., Demos Medical Publishing, 2017

.

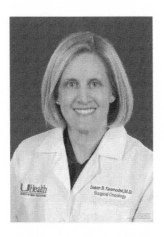

Dr. Kesmodel is an Associate Professor of Surgery in the Division of Surgical Oncology in the DeWitt Daughtry Family Department of Surgery, University of Miami Health System. She graduated from Princeton University with a degree in computer science and received her medical degree from the University of Pennsylvania Perelman School of Medicine. She completed a residency in general surgery at the Hospital of the University of Pennsylvania and a fellowship in surgical oncology at MD Anderson Cancer Center. Dr. Kesmodel serves as the Director of Breast Surgical Oncology and Co-Leader of the Breast Site Disease Group for the Sylvester Comprehensive Cancer Center.

She has written numerous articles on breast cancer management and outcomes and recently helped develop, author and edit a new handbook of breast cancer and breast diseases. She is a member of the Society of Surgical Oncology, American Society of Breast Surgeons, American College of Surgeons, and Association of Academic Surgeons and currently serves on the Publications Committee for the American Society of Breast Surgeons and the Training Committee for the Society of Surgical Oncology. Dr. Kesmodel is also a member of the Breast Committee and the Breast Translational Research Sub-committee for NRG Oncology.

51

4

BREAST CANCER ONCOLOGY: SUBTYPES, STAGING AND CHEMOTHERAPEUTIC AGENTS

CARMEN CALFA, M.D.

I would like to start this chapter by thanking my friend Cindy Papale-Hammontree for the opportunity to participate in writing such an important book. It will help those who read it to understand breast cancer and how to navigate through the maze of diagnosis, treatments, and survivorship issues with knowledge, confidence, and strength for the best outcomes.

Breast cancer is the most frequently diagnosed malignancy, accounting for over 1 million cases each year. It is the leading cause of cancer death in women worldwide. In the United States, breast cancer is the most common female cancer and the second most common cause of cancer death in women. [1] Once the woman/man is diagnosed with breast cancer it is important to understand the extent of disease, the type of breast cancer, and the treatment options.

The first question that usually comes in mind is, "Why did I get breast cancer?" The second one relates to the fear for the children being at increased risk. While there are many risk factors, approximately 60% of patients will not be able to identify the cause; 30% have a family history of breast cancer; and only 5-10% of breast cancer patients contract it because of genetic mutations. Several other genes have been identified recently, and it's important that the family history is obtained accurately from both sides of the families, three generations up. Understanding the factors that could have contributed to the development of breast cancer helps with the evaluation of the risk of developing a secondary event, the risk for additional cancers in the same individual, and the risk for first degree relatives. It also gives an opportunity to correct some of the modifiable risk factors, such as reducing alcohol intake, smoking cessation, increased exercise, improved diet, weight loss, and avoiding hormone replacement therapy, to name a few. Unfortunately, we can't change the fact that we are getting older. But, in the big scheme of things, that's a good thing!

I will try to guide you from the time of diagnosis to understanding the treatment plan and the short and long-term side effects that are associated with the treatment and the disease itself. Being diagnosed with breast cancer is overwhelming and scary. However, keep in mind that this is one of the most curable cancers when detected early.

Also, be aware that there is a lot of information shared by other patients in blogs or social media. While it is good to have a support system and someone to lean on, one should carefully consider the sources. I am hoping that this book will be an excellent resource and prepare you for the consultation with the team of experts that will be involved in your multidisciplinary care.

Breast cancer is a complex disease, one that affects the individual and their family at many levels, for a very long time. I call it the "gift that keeps on giving." From the diagnosis to treatment and survivorship, breast cancer requires a multidisciplinary approach. To achieve an excellent outcome, everyone involved in the care must be outstanding and right.

Now, going back to the diagnosis of breast cancer. The day the person is diagnosed is the day they become a survivor. Whether it's a man or a woman, the steps are the same. Since breast cancer is rare in men, there are no large studies guiding us in the management of male breast cancer. Oncologists extrapolate the information from the studies performed in women until more collaborative research results will be available. Without going into details, any male diagnosed with breast cancer should be offered genetic testing.

Once you, your friend, or your loved ones get through the overwhelming first day, the next step is to reach out for guidance and to set up appointments with the best of the best. My goal for my chapter is that it will inspire anyone who reads it to schedule those appointments for their entire breast cancer treatment journey.

There are several things one needs to know about breast cancer. First, a medical oncologist should always be part of the team. It cannot just be anyone. You want to be seen by a subspecialized breast oncologist if possible. The more patients with the same disease one doctor sees the greater their expertise. In the United States, breast cancer accounts for approximately 266,000 cases each year and is responsible for taking away from us 40,000 women every year [1]. For every 100 women there is 1 man diagnosed with breast cancer. Breast cancer mortality rates have been decreasing since the 1970s [2]. This decrease in mortality is likely due at least in part to improved breast cancer screening (with mammograms) and more effective therapies.

While is tempting to google trying to find the answers, it gets extremely complicated, overwhelming, misleading, and confusing. It takes 10 years to become an oncologist – imagine trying to master that in a few nights. My best advice is to just google the credentials of the doctors you plan to see and, hopefully, by then you have already reached out for this book.

These are the questions you must ask if you are going as the patient, a friend, or a caregiver.

1. What is breast cancer?

2. What are the types of breast cancer?

3. What is the stage of my breast cancer?

4. What is the treatment, when, and for how long?

Let us go one by one.

1. WHAT IS BREAST CANCER

Breast cancer is a disease in which malignant (cancer) cells form in the tissues of the breast due to unregulated growth. Cell division and death are well regulated in our bodies and kept in check by tight sophisticated mechanisms.

If an error occurs in this process, the cell will divide and multiply uncontrollably, leading to cancer growth and potential metastasis to local lymph nodes or distant organs. That is why diagnosing the cancer early is key. Not every breast mass is malignant and not every malignant breast mass is breast cancer. The breast can give rise to other invasive malignancies separate from the primary breast cancer. These tumors are rare and include sarcoma of the breast, Phyllodes tumor, Paget's disease and lymphoma. A qualified pathologist can make the correct diagnosis. In rare instances, the cancer in the breast can be a metastasis coming from another site of the body. This will not be considered "breast cancer" and it will be called by the name of the site where it originates (for example, renal cancer metastatic to the breast).

The breast is made up of lobes and ducts. Each breast has 15-to-20 sections called lobes. Each lobe has many smaller sections called lobules. Lobules end in dozens of tiny bulbs that can make milk. The lobes, lobules, and bulbs are linked by thin tubes called ducts.

The graph below helps you understand the anatomy of the breast.

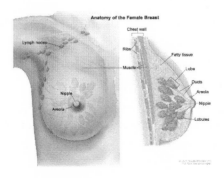

2. TYPES OF BREAST CANCER

Once a piece of the breast cancer is removed, it is analyzed in the lab by a specialized breast pathologist.

There are various histologic types of breast carcinoma that differ in microscopic appearance and biological behavior. The most common types of epithelial breast cancer are infiltrating ductal carcinoma (known as IDC) accounting for 70-80% of the invasive lesions, infiltrating lobular carcinoma(ILC), accounting for about 8% of invasive breast cancer. Mixed ductal/lobular carcinoma at about 7% of invasive breast cancers. Other histologic types include metaplastic, mucinous, tubular, medullary, papillary carcinoma and together they account for less than 5% of the invasive cancers. A rare type is also inflammatory breast cancer which presents as a swollen, erythematous breast with the skin looking like an orange peel. It can mimic an infection and many times an antibiotic is the first step. The key is to consider cancer as a possible diagnosis and if the infection does not resolve after the course of antibiotic, to pursue a diagnostic work up. A negative mammogram does not rule out breast cancer. The same with a negative biopsy.

If things don't make sense, look for answers. The grade of breast cancer characterizes the degree of tumor differentiation. The closer the cells look to the normal breast cells, the lower the grade and the less the aggressiveness.

Now, you want to know why you hear so many patients saying they are on Tamoxifen or another "hormonal pill" and some are not. Some receive Herceptin, and some do not. These indications come from understanding the type of breast cancer when it comes to expression of estrogen and progesterone receptors as well as HER2 protein expression. We call this "prognostic markers" and I would like to make it simple to understand.

Any newly diagnosed breast cancer must be tested for expression of estrogen receptor progesterone receptor and HER2 expression. Soon, we will be adding to this list. This information is critical for therapeutic purposes.

- Estrogen receptors (ER) are a group of proteins found inside cells. They are the receptors that are activated by the hormone estrogen.
- Progesterone receptor (PR) is a protein found inside cells. It is activated by the steroid hormone progesterone.
- Cancer expressing ER PR positivity comprised most of the cases, about 80%.
- HER2 is a protein that in humans is encoded by ERBB2 gene. HER2 is a member of the human epidermal growth factor receptor.

HER2 overexpression is present in 20% of patients. It is detected by uniform intense membrane staining of more than 30% of the invasive tumor cells by immunohistochemistry (IHC 3+) or the presence of HER2 gene amplification by fluorescence in situ hybridization (FISH) defined by a ratio of HER-2/CEP 17 greater or equal to 2.

Amplification or over-expression of this oncogene has been shown to play a crucial role in the development and progression of certain aggressive types of breast cancer. In recent years the protein has become an important biomarker and target of therapy for approximately 20% of breast cancer patients. [3]

If cancer expresses estrogen/progesterone receptor the therapy will include an antiestrogen or estrogen receptor blocker, generically called "hormonal therapy "which is more of a misnomer as, in fact, it defines an "anti-hormonal" therapy. If the HER2 protein is overexpressed/ amplified the tumor is called "Her 2 positive" and the treatment will involve anti-HER2 therapy. I will cover the treatment options in the treatment section below.

As we learn more about breast cancer, we realized that their molecular signature dictate the biological behavior. Gene expression studies allow for the molecular classification of breast cancer into distinct subtypes. These include luminal subtypes, which account for the majority of ER-positive breast cancers, a HER2 enriched subtype, and ER-negative or basal subtypes, which includes most triple-negative breast cancers. Several genomic tests have been developed looking at the molecular signature and defining the cancer biology, predicting a response to certain therapies and having prognostic implications for our patients. Having a correct diagnosis is crucial as the treatment depends on it. You just learned the histological and molecular types of breast cancer and the differential diagnosis for a malignant breast mass.

Now that you received that information, you are ready for question 3.

3. STAGES OF BREAST CANCER

The extent of the disease on presentation defines its stage. It also influences the treatment options, outcomes and the treatment goals.

While patients with stage 0-3 are treated with curative intent and for a limited amount of time, stage 4 involves distant sites, away from the breast and local regional lymph nodes and are considered a "chronic condition" that we are striving to find a cure for. For now, stage 4 is considered incurable; treatment is given with palliative intent, to improve symptoms and quality of life. More and more we are seeing "exceptions to this rule" and patients outlive their initially thought life expectancy due to better treatment options. A growing minority can be considered "cured."

Even when breast cancer is "caught early," the treatment is complex and involves a multidisciplinary approach. Patients ask me often, "I removed both of my breasts because I wanted to be aggressive and never have to worry about it again. Why do I still need chemotherapy if surgery 'took it all out?' How could it 'come back' if I no longer have breasts?" As a breast medical oncologist for more than a decade, I feel that getting the patient to understand why she/he does what she/or does is crucial. Once that happens, the patient and the medical team become motivated partners in the fight against breast cancer.

Unfortunately, breast cancer like many other cancers, is considered a systemic disease on initial presentation. That means that there is a possibility of microscopic disease being present outside of the breast and local regional lymphatic system at the time of the diagnosis. If the disease is detectable by conventional radiological evaluation outside of the breast and the lymph nodes than the disease is considered metastatic or stage 4.

We have the so-called staging system that considers the size of the tumor, the number of lymph nodes involved, and the presence or absence of distant metastatic disease. We call it *TNM staging*: T for tumor, N for lymph, and M for distant metastasis. If the patient presents with disease in the bones, liver, lung, brain, or other organs, the stage is 4, and the patient will likely receive treatment for the rest of her or his life.

T speaks for the size of the tumor and N for the number of lymph nodes. The higher the T and the N the higher the stage.

Now you can imagine that a tiny tumor limited to the breast and not affecting the lymph nodes will be a stage I if smaller than 2 cm. If the tumor is anywhere between 2-5 cm and/or has I-3 positive lymph nodes stage changes to 2, a larger than 5 cm tumor with positive lymph nodes, or even a small tumor with more than 3 positive lymph nodes make a stage 3 and so on.

The stages of invasive cancer are I, 2, 3, and 4.

Stage 0 or ductal carcinoma in situ is a pre-invasive condition that does not require chemotherapy. However, the patient will require surgery, possible radiation, and possible endocrine treatment to prevent further invasive and noninvasive breast cancer.

The determination of the extent of the tumor in the breast and loco regional lymph nodes is done by mammogram, ultrasound, and MRI. This is well covered in the radiology section by my colleague, Dr Monica Yepes.

Women with advanced cases of breast cancer may present with

skin changes (also known as peau d'orange) or axillary adenopathy. Less than five percent of patients present with signs or symptoms of metastatic breast cancer on initial presentation.

But not everyone needs "scans" to look for distant metastatic disease because they are likely to be negative in stage 1 and 2. For patients with early stage breast cancer (stage 1 or 2), a bone scan is indicated if patient has localized bone pain or an elevated alkaline phosphatase (seen on the initial blood work). If the bone scan is negative and clinical suspicion warrants further evaluation, magnetic resonance imaging (MRI) should be performed localized to the symptomatic area.

The same principle applies for CT scan of the liver and/or chest. If abnormal liver function tests, an elevated alkaline phosphatase, abdominal pain, or an abnormal abdominal or pelvic examination, we obtain a computed tomography (CT) scan of the abdomen. Abdominal MRI or ultrasound would be reasonable alternatives, as would positron emission tomography-computed tomography (PET-CT). For patients with stage IIIA or higher disease, regardless of whether symptoms are present or not, we obtain a whole-body PET-CT or, alternatively, a bone scan as well as a CT scan of the chest, abdomen, and pelvis. Patients with inflammatory breast cancer, regardless of stage, should also undergo imaging evaluation.

We recently learned that besides size and number of lymph nodes, the "genomic signature" of a tumor dictates its biological behavior. I will cover this briefly in the treatment section. The most recent staging system incorporates this into the staging. A larger tumor with a low biological risk would be staged lower than a smaller tumor with aggressive biology. This affects the treatment choices and it's an important change to the way we look at the breast cancer stage.

4. TREATMENT OF BREAST CANCER

Treatment of breast cancer requires a multidisciplinary approach. A team of breast cancer specialists – surgical oncologist, medical oncologist, pathologist, and radiation oncologist should get together to review each new case before treatment is performed. This happens during so called "tumor boards" and has the benefit of prospectively and collectively reviewing all breast images, the clinical manifestation, the staging scans, pathology, genetic risk factors, patient preference, and patient-associated medical problems all at the same time. The patient benefits from the opportunity to obtain several expert opinions at once. Treatment is personalized and tailored to one's breast cancer specifics. We like to say "one size does not fit all" because it doesn't.

This is how we look at each case.

If the patient is relatively healthy, we treat the younger and older similarly. We review the images and the pathology as well as the staging work up. **If we decide the breast cancer is localized** (stage 1-3), the treatment components are:

Surgery to remove the cancer. It's important that the cancer is not at the margin. Just like when you clean an apple of a bad spot, you go around until you find healthy tissue to minimize the risk of the cancer returning in that place. Since breast cancer can travel via lymphatics and blood stream to lymph nodes, it's important that we address the lymph nodes in the axilla surgically as well. We have made progress and moved away from removing the entire breast and all the lymph nodes in everyone; we are now able to select those we can have the cancer removed, while preserving the breast and most lymph nodes. This is covered at length by my colleague, Dr. Susan Kesmodel, in the surgical chapter.

The chances of curing a patient from breast cancer are equal with a mastectomy vs. lumpectomy and radiation.

What determines the overall outcome is the stage of the cancer, the biology of the cancer, and responsiveness to **medical treatment** (so-called "systemic therapy").

As I mentioned before, breast cancer is a "systemic disease," meaning microscopic disease can be present far from the cancer at the time of diagnosis. Detecting that microscopic disease will allow us to monitor the treatment effect and know "what we are going after." Research is being done to identify either the circulating tumor cells or their free DNA in the blood stream as a surrogate for the "microscopic disease". At present, once a cancer is removed, we deliver systemic therapy "blindly", without being able to evaluate response to therapy. Not every patient will have microscopic disease but because we can't identify with certainty those who do, we are overtreating many of our patients. If the disease never recurs we know our treatment was effective.

Once the cancer is removed surgically, we can precisely evaluate the prognostic markers ER PR HER2, grade, rate of proliferation or growth (measured by KI 67) as well as the pathological stage.

The medical treatment given after surgery for stage 1-3 is called "adjuvant."

If tumors are larger than 5 cm and /or the involved lymph nodes are greater than 3, patient will be recommended to receive chemotherapy. For smaller tumors and fewer positive lymph nodes, we use the biological "score" only if the tumor is ER positive HER2 negative. If HER2 is amplified, the patient will most likely be recommended anti-HER2 treatment to be added to chemotherapy and continue after chemotherapy is completed for a total of 1-2 years. I will elaborate on anti HER2 agents in the curative portion of this chapter. If the ER and PR are positive, hormonal therapy, also called endocrine therapy, will be given for 5-10 years.

If the cancer is lacking ER PR and HER2 (triple negative) we don t have a specific target and chemotherapy is indicating for tumors as small as 6mm in size. In addition to ER PR HER2, lymph node status and size, for early stage ER+Her2 negative, we use genomic testing to identify risk of distant recurrence and benefit from chemotherapy.

The emergence of genomics techniques and the ability to simultaneously measure the expression of thousands of genes has led to the identification of biology-based prognostic profiles, several of which have been validated and are in clinical use. While Oncotype Dx Recurrence Score (RS) is the most well-validated, MammaPrint, EndoPredict®, Predictor Analysis of Microarray 50 (PAM50), and the Breast Cancer Index may also be used.

Again, there are several genomic tests available and we apply them depending on the clinical situation.

For instance, a patient with 1-3 positive lymph nodes ER/PR positive and HER2 negative breast cancer used to be considered "clinically high risk" and chemotherapy was indicated. After conducting a large randomized study, we learned that if the 70 gene signature dictated by MammaPrint is low, the patient will do very well in the absence of chemotherapy. Moreover, chemotherapy will not increase the chances of staying cancer-free. In this case, chemotherapy could be avoided, and the patient will derive great benefit from endocrine therapy. Conversely, if the MammaPrint indicates a "high risk" biology, the risk of distant recurrence is high, and this could be lowered significantly by using chemotherapy. [7]

In a patient with a cancer size 6 mm to 5 cm, with negative lymph nodes, ER/PR positive HER2 negative, the decision to use chemotherapy was traditionally made by looking at the patient's age, size, and grade of the tumor. Now we have data to forgo chemotherapy in patients with low or intermediate risk genomic scores (RS ≤25) measured by 21 gene Oncotype Dx. We can also predict risk of distant recurrence and benefit of chemotherapy and for high risk tumors chemotherapy greatly reduces the risk of recurrence, therefore we strongly recommend it.

There are situations when we recommend chemotherapy with or without anti-HER2 therapy or hormonal therapy to be given before surgery. In this case the treatment is "neoadjuvant"

There are several advantages to this approach.

1. The tumor is still in the body; therefore, we can assess treatment effectiveness
2. We can shrink the tumor and the lymph nodes, minimizing the amount of tissue that needs to be removed at the time of surgery, potentially increasing one's chance of preserving her breast and decreasing the chance of lymphedema.
3. If the therapy is not effective it could be aborted before completion and alternative therapies can be tried.
4. It allows to start earlier and prevents delays potentially caused by surgical complications
5. It allows testing the tumor response at the time of surgery, molecular sequencing and exploration of new drugs that potentially can increase the cure rates. Significant research is being conducted in this field.

My preference: If the treatment option is clear and we have all the information we need to decide prior to surgery, I prefer to give systemic therapy upfront. It's a "cleaner," "faster," and more informative approach that allows less extensive surgery and potentially less radiation.

Upon reviewing the case in tumor board, the disease could be found that is spread to distant organs up front. **This is called "de novo stage 4."** If the patient was treated before for a localized disease and later presents with distant metastasis, it is considered **recurrent metastatic breast cancer, stage 4.** Breast cancer favors bones, liver, lung, brain and other sites. While HER2 positive cancer favors the brain, ER positive breast cancer favors the bones. [8]

Many times, the metastatic sites will cause symptoms. The treatment goal becomes palliation of symptoms and improvement in survival. Surgery of the primary site in the breast is no longer recommended in the majority of the cases and the focus becomes finding the systemic disease that will control the disease everywhere. We learned that the tumor can be "heterogeneous" and differences can be appreciated within the same tumor or between the primary tumor and the metastatic site. [9]

The tumor cell has several mechanisms of growth, division, and metastasis and it quickly changes to develops new pathways that will confer resistance to therapies. The initial treatments have higher chances of being effective and the responses are usually longer. As we change from one line of therapy to another (one agent to another) resistance tends to develop, the treatments tend to be less effective, and shorter-lasting. We do lose more than 40, 000 women to breast cancer per year in the United States and research is ongoing to elucidate mechanism of resistance, find new therapies, and engage the immune system in a meaningful way by using immunotherapies and modify the lifestyle factors that could have a negative impact in the outcome.

Depending on the prognostic markers, the volume of the disease, and the involment of vital organs the patient will be recommended to start therapy. Survival of a patient with stage 4 is on average 5 years.

If she/he has triple negative breast cancer (TNBC) conventional treatmnet will involve chemotherapy. Different "targets" are explored and new therapies are developed.

If patient has ER+HER2 negative disease treatmnet will involve hormonal therapy as well as chemotehrapy.

If patient has ER/PR+HER2 positive disease treatment will involve chemotherapy, anti HER2 therapy, hormonal therapy. Most of the time we sequence drugs to avoid overlaping toxicity and asure longer duration of available drugs.

New approaches have been adding a new class of CDK4/6 inhibitors, mTor inhibitors, HDAC inhitors to endocrine therapy. This has kept patients in a disease control state twice as long compared to hormonal therapy alone for a minimal added toxicity. The art of oncology is to use only as much " force" as you need to supress the cancer.

Below is a picture that depicts the breast cancer intricated molecular pathways. [10]

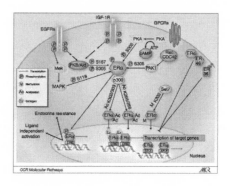

Hopefully I made clear the principles of systemic therapy. Now I will elaborate on specifics of hormonal therapy, anti HER2 therapy, and chemotherapy.

Again, in stage 1-3 the treatment is given over a limited period. Chemotherapy options range from 12 weeks to 20 weeks. Anti-HER2 therapy is given for 1-2 years. Hormonal therapy is given for 5-10 years. The decision is made after serious multidisciplinary evaluation by the team of experts with the patient's goals in mind.

In stage 4, treatment is "chronic" for the duration of one's life and involves systemic and local options, depending on the type of breast cancer.

HORMONAL THERAPY

Cancer that express estrogen or progesterone receptor use estrogen to stimulate the cell proliferation and metastasis.

Blocking either the receptors (estrogen receptor blockers), the estrogen production in the ovaries (chemical or surgical menopause) or in other tissue (aromatase inhibitors) is an effective way to deprive the cell of the estrogen needed in the signaling pathway.

The approved treatment choices are listed below. Tamoxifen is indicated in premenopausal female or postmenopausal patients who cannot tolerate an aromatase inhibitor.

Aromatase inhibitors are recommended for postmenopausal female.

Selective estrogen receptor modulators, called SERMs, block the effects of estrogen in the breast tissue. SERMs work by sitting in the estrogen receptors in breast cells, therefore estrogen is not able to attach to the cell and signal the cell's growth and multiplication. Cells in other tissues in the body, such as bones and the uterus, also have estrogen receptors but they are slightly different. SERMs are "selective", with dual function, they block estrogen's action in breast cells and activate estrogen's action in other cells including bone, liver, and uterine cells, hence their side effect profile will reflect that.

There are three SERMs: tamoxifen (also called tamoxifen citrate; brand name: Nolvadex); tamoxifen in liquid form (brand name: Soltamox), Evista (chemical name: raloxifene), Fareston (chemical name: toremifene).While the most common side effects of this drugs are fatigue, hot flashes, night sweats, vaginal discharge, mood swings, they rarely can cause life threatening side effects including blood clots, strokes, and endometrial cancer.

Another group of endocrine therapy are the Estrogen receptor down-regulators, called ERD. They block the effects of estrogen in breast tissue in a similar manner with SERM, but they also reduce the number of estrogen receptors and change the shape of breast cell estrogen receptors, so their function is altered.

While research is ongoing to add an oral ERD, currently Fulvestrant (Faslodex) is the only ERD available to treat hormone-receptor-positive breast cancer and it's approved only in postmenopausal women with advanced breast cancer disease.

Aromatase inhibitors stop the production of estrogen in post-menopausal women by blocking the enzyme that is needed to convert androgen into small amounts of estrogen in the body. They are approved in postmenopausal women with early or advanced disease.

There are three aromatase inhibitors: Arimidex (chemical name: anastrozole), Aromasin (chemical name: exemestane), Femara (chemical name: letrozole)

Research has shown that removing estrogen or blocking estrogen receptors is an effective way to shrink estrogen sensitive tumors or to decrease recurrences in those treated with surgery for an estrogen sensitive breast cancer. The first observation was made in animals in1896 and Tamoxifen was approved by the Food and Drug Administration (FDA) in 1977 for treatment of metastatic breast cancer. [11]

Studies have compared different strategies of estrogen manipulation. The endocrine therapy "intensity" goes up as we move away from tamoxifen to an aromatase inhibitor with or without ovarian suppression. The side effects caused by the lack of estrogen increase as well.

In a premenopausal female the main source of estrogen are the ovaries. Their function can be blocked chemically with an injection given subcutaneously either monthly or every 3 months. The 2 drugs approved are Zoladex (Goserelin) and Triptorelin (Triptodur). Blocking the ovarian function chemically is known as Ovarian Suppression. (OS) and it's associated with postmenopausal side effects, as expected.

Depending on the risk of recurrence or the stage of disease the endocrine therapy recommended will range from Tamoxifen to Tamoxifen and Ovarian Suppression or Aromatase inhibitors with without ovarian suppression.

The duration of treatment will also range from 5-10 years in the curative setting (stage 1-3) and will vary widely in stage IV.

Aromatase inhibitors are associated with musculoskeletal disease, bone loss, hot flushes, dyslipidemia, bone loss, vaginal changes, decreased sexual function and others. They are not associated with endometrial cancer and the risk of blood clots is minuscule.

For postmenopausal women with estrogen sensitive breast cancer treated with curative intent research has shown that adding a bone modifying agent (such as Fosomax, Boniva , Zometa, or Prolia) is beneficial in decreasing bone events as well the chance of breast cancer recurrence.

You will be alarmed hearing about the risk of osteonecrosis of the jaw with this drug; however, the risk is minimal when dental evaluation and clearance is done beforehand.

ANTI-HER2 THERAPY

Cancer cells from a tissue sample can be tested to see which genes are normal and abnormal Genes encode the recipes for the various proteins needed for a normal cell function and cycle.

HER2 (human epidermal growth factor receptor 2) is one such gene that can play a role in the development of breast cancer. The *HER2* gene is also called the *ERBB2 (Erb-B2 receptor tyrosine kinase 2)* gene.

The *HER2* gene makes HER2 proteins that are receptors on breast cells. If the gene makes too many copies of itself and receptors are overexpressed, this leads to cell grows and uncontrollable division.

Like explained before, breast cancers with *HER2* gene amplification or HER2 protein overexpression are called HER2-positive and they represent 20-25% of the breast cancers. The anti-HER2 therapy had revolutionized the treatment options for this type of cancers and their prognosis. In the curative setting it had decreased the chance of recurrence and the chance of dying from this disease by half.

In the metastatic setting it had doubled the time the patients live with the disease.

Research has shown that some breast cancers that are HER2-positive can become HER2-negative over time. Likewise, a HER2-negative breast cancer can become HER2-positive over time. In case of a recurrence, a biopsy is needed to verify prognostic markers and HER2 status. It's also recommended during the stage 4 disease, at different phases of progression.

The first anti-HER2 monoclonal antibody was Trastuzumab (Herceptin), approved in 1998. Since then, additional anti-HER2 agents were added to the portfolio and they are given in different combinations depending on the stage of the disease.

I will briefly list the approved drugs, but many new ones are in different research phases and they will soon gain FDA approval.

Herceptin (chemical name: trastuzumab), which works against HER2-positive breast cancers by blocking the ability of the cancer cells to receive chemical signals that tell the cells to grow.

Tykerb (chemical name: lapatinib) was approved in 2008 for stage 4 disease and it works against HER2-positive breast cancers by blocking certain proteins that can cause uncontrolled cell growth.

Kadcyla (chemical name: T-DM1 or ado-trastuzumab emtansine), approved in 2013 for stage 4 disease is a combination of Herceptin and the chemotherapy medicine emtansine. Kadcyla was designed to deliver emtansine to cancer cells in a targeted way by attaching emtansine to Herceptin. Herceptin then carries emtansine to the HER2-positive cancer cells.

Perjeta (chemical name: pertuzumab) was approved in 2013 for early and late stage. Similar to Herceptin, Perjeta works against HER2-positive breast cancers by blocking the cancer cells' ability to receive growth signals.

Nerlynx (chemical name: neratinib), approved for early and late stage in 2018, fights HER2-positive breast cancers by blocking the cancer cells' ability to receive growth signals.

The sequence duration and combination with other anti her agents as well as chemotherapy is personalized depending patients characteristics and stage of disease. The additional drugs discovered after Herceptin had improved the prognosis of this cancer types further.

CHEMOTHERAPY

Chemotherapy treatment uses medicine to weaken and destroy cancer cells in the body, including cells at the original cancer site and any cancer cells that may have spread to another part of the body. Chemotherapy is a systemic therapy that affects the entire body by going through the bloodstream.

There are quite a few chemotherapy medicines. In many cases, a combination of two or more medicines will be used as chemotherapy treatment for breast cancer in the curative setting while single agents are mostly preferred in the advanced, metastatic phase.

Chemotherapy is used to treat early stage BC as well as metastatic disease.

Their main side effects include nausea, vomiting, diarrhea/constipation, change in taste, lack of appetite, change in weight (up or down), nail toxicity, neuropathy, skin changes, infertility and very rarely antracyclines can cause cardiotoxicity and secondary myelodysplasia or leukemia.

Most of the toxicities can be managed with supportive medication. The way I look at it is that chemotherapy can prevent a recurrence and can save one's life. Risk and benefit has to be weighted and discussed specifically with every individual patient. There are not 2 patients with identical risk/benefit ratio. That is where the art of oncology comes in to offer every patient the regimen that she/he would benefit the most. This cytotoxic agents act at different cell level and they have different side effect profiles therefore a patient with, for example, neuropathy from diabetes will be given the less neurotoxic chemotherapeutic agent.

Some of the most effective and commonly used agents/combinations are

AC: Adriamycin and Cytoxan

AT: Adriamycin and Taxotere

CMF: Cytoxan, methotrexate, and fluorouracil

FAC: fluorouracil, Adriamycin, and Cytoxan

CAF: Cytoxan, Adriamycin, and fluorouracil

(The FAC and CAF regimens use the same medicines but use different doses and frequencies)

Eribulin (Halaven)

Gemcitabin (Gemzar)

Ixabepilon (Ixempra)

Carboplatinum/Cisplatinum (Platinum agents)

Vinorelbine (Navelbine)

Capecitabine (Xeloda)
Paclitaxel (Taxol)
Nab-paclitaxel (Abraxane)
Peg-doxorubicin (Doxil)

In HER2 positive disease anti-HER2 drugs can be added to different chemotherapy agents depending on the stage of disease.

ANTI CDK4/6

When we looked at the cancer cell "map" [6] and see its complexity we understand why eradicating cancer is difficult. Through different pathways, mechanisms of resistance occur.

New class of medication have been recently approved to enhance endocrine sensitivity and help patients with advanced, estrogen positive breast cancer stay twice as long in remission when compared to endocrine therapy alone. They belong to the class knows as 'anti CDK4/6". 3 agents are available:
Palbociclib (Ibrance)
Ribociclib (Kisquali)
Abemaciclib (Verzenio)

MTOR Inhibitors

Everolimus (Afinitor) in combination with endocrine therapy has also shown to improve the time patient's disease is controlled and it's approved for stage 4 ER positive disease.

PARP Inhibitors

The PARP (poly ADP-ribose polymerase) enzyme fixes DNA damage in cells, including DNA damage caused by chemotherapy medicines. Scientists developed PARP inhibitors based on the idea that a medicine that interferes with or inhibits the PARP enzyme might make it harder for cancer cells to fix damaged DNA, which could make chemotherapy more effective. In 2018, the U.S. Food and Drug Administration (FDA) approved Lynparza (chemical name: olaparib) as the first PARP inhibitor to treat breast cancer. Lynparza is used to treat metastatic, HER2-negative breast cancer in women with a *BRCA1* or *BRCA2* mutation that has been previously treated with chemotherapy.

IMMUNOTHERAPIES

Immunotherapy medicines use the power of our own's body immune system to attack cancer cells. Immunotherapy medicines work by helping the immune system work harder and smarter to attack cancer cells.

Different strategies have been tried over the last decade. The problem is that the cancer "flies under the radar" when it comes to the immune system recognition. Vaccine therapies meant to stimulate the recognition of the cancer cells by the immune system while "checkpoint inhibitors" unleash the immune system allowing it to go after the cancer cells. They are in advanced research phases for the treatment of early as well as advanced breast cancer.

CLINICAL TRIALS IN BREAST CANCER

While several clinical trials are ongoing, the theme of conquering breast cancer in 2018 has been evolving around "precision medicine "and use of "immunotherapy".

VACCINE THERAPY

Vaccine therapies for breast cancer treatment are designed to help the immune system recognize the cancer cells as a threat and mount a response. Like traditional vaccines, these vaccines are generally made from weakened or dead breast cancer cells — either patient's own or those cultivated in a laboratory. The hope is that once the immune system becomes aware of the antigens in the vaccine, it responds by making antibodies. These antibodies could then attack and destroy any remaining cancer cells. The immune system builds memory and later, if any new cancer cells appear, the circulating antibodies would destroy them also. Several vaccine therapies are ongoing for early and late stage of breast cancer.

CHECK POINT INHIBITORS

To start an immune system response to a foreign invader, the immune system must be able to distinguish between cells or substances that are "self" (part of you) versus "non-self" (not part of you and possibly harmful).

Some of these proteins that help your immune system recognize "self" cells are called immune checkpoints. Cancer cells sometimes find ways to use these immune checkpoint proteins as a shield to avoid being identified and attacked by the immune system.

Immune checkpoint inhibitors target these immune checkpoint proteins and help the immune system recognize and attack cancer cells. Immune checkpoint inhibitors essentially take the brakes off the immune system by blocking checkpoint inhibitor proteins on cancer cells or on the T cells that respond to them.

The most advanced agents belong to PD-1/PD-L1 and CTLA-4 inhibitors groups.

Keytruda (chemical name: pembrolizumab), approved for other cancers, is in advanced research phase for breast cancer and approved for a subset of triple negative breast cancer. [12]

Opdivo (chemical name: nivolumab), approved for other cancers, is in research phase for breast cancer in combination with other agents.

Tecentriq (chemical name: atezolizumab), Bavencio (chemical name: avelumab), Imfinzi (chemical name: durvalumab) use to treat other cancers, they are in research phase for breast cancer.

Yervoy (chemical name: ipilimumab) targets the CTLA-4 protein and pushes the T cells to become activated to attack cancer cells.

One big concern about immune checkpoint inhibitor medicines is that they may allow the immune system to attack some healthy cells and organs as the medicines essentially take the brakes off the immune system. The T cells may start attacking cells other than cancer cells and this can be associated with some serious side effects include problems with the lungs, liver, intestines, pancreas, and kidneys.

CONCLUSION

I am a passionate breast medical oncologist. I am an optimist. I see the half glass full.

I strive to educate unaffected individuals as much as I educate those challenged by breast cancer.

I think "knowledge is power," and that teaming up with experts in the field gives one the best chance to cure breast cancer.

Unfortunately, it's not always pretty and pink. We still loose dear ones to breast cancer. When it gets hard my advice is to stay focused. Just like if you were to cross a big frightening river on a rope, high above it, don't look down. Put one foot in front of the other and look forward.

Through research we got were we are. We are saving most of those diagnosed with breast cancer.

New research can help us find the cure. Stay focused! Set your goals and your priorities. Make a team with your doctor and let her/him know how you feel.

I wish I could share everything in this chapter, but it was not possible. However, I can always be found for questions or advice at the University of Miami Sylvester Comprehensive Cancer Center. The number is (954)-210-1167 or (305) 901-0201.

1. Cancer statistics, 2018.Siegel RL, Miller KD, Jemal A, CA Cancer J Clin. 2018; 68(1):7. Epub 2018 Jan 4.

2. Annual Report to the Nation on the Status of Cancer, 1975-2011, Featuring Incidence of Breast Cancer Subtypes by Race/Ethnicity, Poverty, and State. Kohler BA, Sherman RL, Howlader N, Jemal A, Ryerson AB, Henry KA, Boscoe FP, Cronin KA, Lake A, Noone AM, Henley SJ, Eheman CR, Anderson RN, Penberthy L, J Natl Cancer Inst. 2015;107(6):djv048. Epub 2015 Mar 30.

3. *Mitri Z, Constantine T, O'Regan R (2012).* "The HER2 Receptor in Breast Cancer: Pathophysiology, Clinical Use, and New Advances in Therapy". *Chemotherapy Research and Practice. 2012: 743193*

4. Prognostic significance of Nottingham histologic grade in invasive breast carcinoma.Rakha EA, El-Sayed ME, Lee AH, Elston CW, Grainge MJ, Hodi Z, Blamey RW, Ellis IO J Clin Oncol. 2008; 26(19):3153.

5. A multigene assay to predict recurrence of tamoxifen-treated, node-negative breast cancer.Paik S, Shak S, Tang G, Kim C, Baker J, Cronin M, Baehner FL, Walker MG, Watson D, Park T, Hiller W, Fisher ER, Wickerham DL, Bryant J, Wolmark N N Engl J Med. 2004;351(27):2817. Epub 2004 Dec 10.

6. [Estrogen Receptor Mutations and Changes in Downstream Gene Expression and Signaling Ines Barone, Lauren Brusco and Suzanne A.W. Fuqua

7. 70-Gene Signature as an Aid to Treatment Decisions in Early-Stage Breast Cancer, Fatima Cardoso, M.D., Laura J. van't Veer, Ph.D., Jan Bogaerts, Ph.D.,

8. Metastatic patterns of breast cancer subtypes: What radiologists should know in the era of personalized cancer medicine S.A.Chikarmane[ab] S.H.Tirumani[ab] S.A.Howard[ab] J.P.Jagannathan[ab] P.J.DiPiro[ab]

9. Tumor Heterogeneity in Breast Cancer <u>Gulisa Turashvili</u> and <u>Edi Brogi</u>

10. Estrogen Receptor Mutations and Changes in Downstream Gene Expression and Signaling Ines Barone, Lauren Brusco and Suzanne A.W. Fuqua

11. Breast Cancer Res Treat. 1988 Jul;11(3):197-209.The development of tamoxifen for breast cancer therapy: a tribute to the late Arthur L. Walpole. Jordan VC

12. Adams S, Schmid P, Rugo HS, et al. Phase 2 study of pembrolizumab (pembro) monotherapy for previously treated metastatic triple-negative breast cancer (mTNBC): KEYNOTE-086 cohort A. *J Clin Oncol* 35, 2017 (suppl; abstr 1008)..

≈

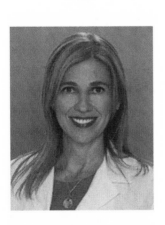

Carmen Calfa, M.D. is a triple board-certified breast medical oncologist and has been recognized for her clinical care and research. She is an assistant professor of clinical medicine at the University of Miami Miller School of Medicine. At Sylvester, Dr. Calfa works as part of a multidisciplinary team of breast cancer experts and researchers. She earned her medical degree from the University of Medicine and Pharmacy of Tirgu-Mures from Romania. Dr. Calfa's career highlights include:

- Research focused on immunotherapy, HER2-positive, and triple negative breast cancers
- Work with underserved women in the tri-county area using unique strategies to increase screening and early detection of breast cancers
- Completed Internal Medicine Residency and Fellowship Training in Hematology Oncology at the University of Miami School of Medicine
- Authored widely published studies

5

BREAST CANCER RADIATION THERAPY 2018

BEATRIZ E. AMENDOLA, MD FACR FASTRO FACRO

Radiation therapy or radiotherapy (RT) is one of the three (3) pillars in the treatment of cancer together with surgery and medical oncology. It uses ionizing radiation to kill malignant cells. Radiotherapy after breast conserving surgery (BCS) has been shown to reduce the risk of breast cancer (BC) recurrence. Younger women tend to have tumors that are more aggressive and have higher risks of recurrence than older women. The reason(s) why younger women do not receive or are not made aware of this treatment is not well known. The literature does not provide concrete answers. Notwithstanding, in 2013, studies found that patients fifty (50) years or younger were less likely to receive radiation therapy (RT) than those in older age brackets. They also found that a woman was less likely to receive RT if she had at least one (1) child less than seven (7) years old, compared with women who had older or no children. Other factors such as health insurance, receiving BCS further from home or in an outpatient setting, as well as living in a region with a lower education level, could be potential barriers to receiving RT at any age. The association between young children and lower utilization of RT was statistically significant only for women aged 20-50 years.

Why women should not be reluctant to receive treatment

Radiotherapy (RT) plays an integral role in the definitive treatment of breast cancer by reducing the risk of locoregional disease recurrence and breast cancer death. Numerous randomized medical research trials have established the success equivalence of breast conservation therapy, composed of: lumpectomy (surgery) followed by local RT as an alternative to mastectomy. Recent data has suggested breast cancer survival benefits with breast conservation therapy. However, despite the literature, current trends show that the percentage of women who elect to undergo mastectomy continues to rise. Moreover, registry data indicate that adjuvant RT is underused after mastectomy in populations with potential established benefits. Fears and misconceptions regarding RT have been identified by both breast surgeons and patients as factors influencing why a patient would choose mastectomy over breast conservation therapy. Interviews of women about their initial feelings regarding RT commonly found descriptions involving fear and anxiety. The majority of patients were also found to have little or no baseline understanding of RT, regardless of sociodemographic factors. A few patients identify RT as a "modern" cancer treatment, suggesting that perceptions of RT have not kept up with the significant advances in the field. In conclusion, fears and misconceptions regarding RT contribute to its underuse.

Despite the wealth of published literature evaluating the efficacy and toxicity outcomes of breast RT, there is relatively little known regarding the patient's perspective concerning their experience with breast RT. In reality, significant advances in breast RT over the last two (2) decades have resulted in increased accuracy, reduced toxicities, and improved treatment convenience.

Additionally, the actual experiences which were recorded were overwhelmingly superior to initial expectations, and the majority of patients agreed that their fears and negative impressions regarding breast RT were unfounded. Recently published studies have shed some light on the reasons why women might avoid radiation therapy in spite of the data proving positive results. If used correctly, this data can play a critical role in counseling patients and healthcare providers on breast radiation therapy. New technologies and better delivery techniques in the management of breast cancer have shown that radiation is safe and has minimal toxicity associated with the treatment.

Early Stage Breast Cancer

In early breast cancer, where there are no genetic factors that can change the course of the disease, we can obtain 95% cure rates with modern radiation therapy while patients are able to conserve their breast. Breast conservation treatment (BCT) is the preferred method for the overwhelming majority of women who present with early stage breast cancer. It consists of a minimally-invasive surgery which removes the primary tumor most often called a partial or segmental mastectomy (synonyms: lumpectomy, tylectomy, tumorectomy, quadrantectomy) followed by adjuvant radiation therapy (RT) to the whole breast. The addition of RT to conserving surgery is necessary because, as shown in multiple studies, it reduces the risk of local recurrence and results in an absolute improvement in overall survival of 5-7% at 15 years compared to surgery alone. So why do we keep seeing so many women go for mastectomies, with possibility of severe complications when we now have definitive data supporting otherwise? Could it be the vanity and the enticement of getting a tummy-tuck and a breast augmentation at the same time? Advances in plastic surgery promise more attractive artificial breasts than years ago. Unfortunately, we do not think about the potential drawbacks of such a drastic approach, such as an increased risk of recurrence and the chance of surgical complications.

Treating the Patient as a Whole

Breast cancer is a systemic disease, not a local one. In other words, it is a disease of the entire body. This is one of the reasons why it is necessary to use some form of systemic hormones or chemotherapy to prevent the tumor from spreading to other areas of the body. For a small number of women, bilateral mastectomies are necessary because they have multicentric disease (cancer in multiple breasts quadrants) or they carry genetic mutations such as BRCA 1 or 2, most commonly seen in women of Ashkenazi Jewish heritage. These cases typically result in an increased lifetime risk of breast cancer in the 65-85% range. However, most double mastectomies are done on the breast with cancer, in addition to a prophylactic (preventative) mastectomy of the healthy breast; even to women without known genetic mutations. There are many scenarios in which the decision to proceed with bilateral mastectomies is based upon fear and an inaccurate assessment of the complete lists of risks and benefits that this option means for a woman with breast cancer. Clearly, a major factor affecting us today is "the Angelina Jolie effect" which remains popular after so many years. She made her BRCA1 gene mutation public in 2013 when she detailed her path to a bilateral mastectomy after learning that this mutation carries an 85% risk for developing breast cancer. However, the BRAC1/2 genes linked to breast cancer are rare (0.25%). In the USA, only one in 800 women in the general population is affected by this genetic mutation.

Present-day cancer guidelines discourage bilateral mastectomies for most women and recommend it only be considered on a case-by-case basis. It is important for women to always get a second opinion and discuss the options with several specialists. Breast cancer treatment calls for a multidisciplinary team approach involving: 1) the breast surgeon, 2) the radiation oncologist and 3) the medical oncologist. Then, you can make an educated decision. When shopping for a new car or clothing or shoes, women compare and 'shop around'. Yet when dealing with breast cancer, most women see only one surgeon and perhaps a plastic surgeon without getting a second opinion. I encourage patients to shop around! It also helps to talk to other women who are going through or have gone through similar experiences and are able to share their thoughts, feelings and options.

Much success has been achieved in curing breast cancer with less aggressive treatments for many years. As noted above, those treatments consist mostly of lumpectomy followed by radiation. There have been many advances in the field of radiation oncology for breast cancer patients. Below are two of the most advanced forms of radiation treatment available, although they may not yet be available at all medical centers nationally.

Radiation Treatment Advances

Accelerated Partial Breast Irradiation (APBI) Brachytherapy: Early Disease

Brachytherapy, derived from the Greek term for "close", indicates placing a radioactive treatment source near or inside the tumor. The advantage is the quick dose fall-off, sparing adjacent tissues from radiation while providing high focal doses on the tumor itself. High dose rate brachytherapy (HDR) refers to the delivery of a high dose of radiation in a relatively short time. The pathways to the insertion of the radioactive source are usually created using catheters inserted into the tumor bed. The radioactive source is inserted at any time post-surgery therefore; it is called an "after loader" technique. Due to the high activity, the source is inserted remotely into the patient using a remote after-loading unit and removed carefully following the completion of treatment.

Accelerated Partial Breast Irradiation (APBI) using HDR is a remotely controlled radiation protocol that treats only the part of the breast which needs it. It is a shorter course of treatment (usually 5 to 7 days), as opposed to conventional external radiation treatment which usually requires 5 to 6 weeks of daily radiation treatments. This treatment delivers radiation to the area where it is needed most with minimal radiation exposure to the adjacent normal tissues which reduces the potential for side effects. APBI can be delivered via the following various techniques: interstitial brachytherapy, which is the oldest method, intracavitary brachytherapy, 3-dimensional (3D) conformal external beam radiation therapy (EBRT), and intraoperative radiation therapy (IORT). PBI has commonly been delivered in more than 5 days, twice daily in 10 fractions. This has drastically decreased the length of treatment from 6 weeks to 1 week. Interstitial brachytherapy requires inserting temporary catheters into the surgical cavity and surrounding tissue to deliver high-dose-rate brachytherapy. Intraoperative radiotherapy (IORT) is used at the time of surgery and delivers RT to the surgical cavity before the surgeon closes the wound during lumpectomy surgery. This can be done in the operating room or by physically moving the patient from the operating room with an open wound to the radiation machine before wound closure. A disadvantage of IORT is that final pathology and margin status are not available at the time of the radiation procedure. In general, APBI represents an alternative to conventional external irradiation for early breast cancer.

Brachytherapy treatment offers several advantages when compared to the traditional external-beam radiation therapy:

- Radiation only targets the area surrounding the tumor bed (after removal of the tumor by surgical lumpectomy) rather than the whole breast.
- Radiation is delivered in fewer treatments at larger doses, so the total number of treatments is usually in only 5-7 days. The fewer number of days required for treatment is especially helpful for patients who live far away from the radiation center or have a busy schedule.
- Elderly women are excellent candidates, because all patients are treated with a shorter course of radiation on an outpatient basis.
- The cosmetic results are excellent.
- Most women feel little or no discomfort during the treatment.

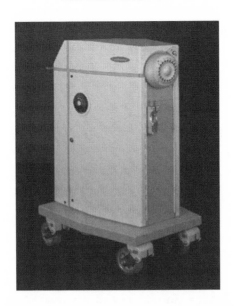

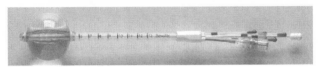

Different radiation therapy schedules using fewer treatments with higher doses of radiation but equivalent to the longer radiation schemes are called hypofractionated radiation, reducing the number of weeks but not the dose of radiation. A hypofractionated radiation schedule is appealing to doctors and patients receiving radiation due to its convenience. Arranging daily trips to get treatment can be a problem for some women so fewer treatment days or a shorter period of time can prove easier to schedule resulting in more women completing all of the recommended radiation therapy treatment sessions.

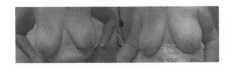

In 2011, the American Society for Radiation Oncology (ASTRO)

released guidelines on hypofractionated whole-breast radiation (PDF) and stated that the technique was as safe and effective as conventional whole-breast radiation for early-stage breast cancer after lumpectomy, for women who meet the four criteria below:

- Fifty years-of-age or older when diagnosed with breast cancer
- Early cancer: stage T1 to T2, no cancer cells have been found in the lymph nodes
- The cancer has been removed with lumpectomy
- The patient is not being administered chemotherapy

Some doctors are still reluctant to use a hypofractionated radiation schedule. Research from the University of Texas MD Anderson Cancer Center randomly assigned 287 women diagnosed with early-stage breast cancer to one of two radiation schedules after lumpectomy:

1. Conventional treatment schedule with a total dose of 50 Gy given in 25 treatments plus a boost dose (149 women)
2. Hypofractionated schedule of a total of 42.56 Gy given in 16 treatments plus a boost dose (138 women)

All the women were age 40 or older and 76% were overweight or obese based on their body mass index. The researchers collected information on how the women viewed the cosmetic and functional outcomes of the radiation treatment, as well as other quality of life factors before the study started, and then at 6 months, 1 year, 2 years, and 3 years after radiation treatment ended. The two radiation schedules had the same outcomes before the study started and at 6 months, 1 year, and 3 years after the treatment ended. Two years after treatment, women in the hypofractionated radiation group reported slightly better functional outcomes than women in the conventional schedule radiation group. This difference was small, but it was statistically significant. This means that the difference in functionality was probably because of the different radiation schedules and not just due to chance. The results of this study echo earlier results showing that hypofractionated radiation is as effective as a conventional radiation schedule. Therefore, hypofractionated treatment, used for the appropriate patients, is a suitable alternative to conventional therapy.

Over the last several decades, it has been questioned whether or not whole breast irradiation is necessary after a lumpectomy for early stage breast cancer. Conventional whole breast irradiation requires a total of 6-6.5 weeks of TX. Hypofractionated whole breast radiation regimens deliver the same dose in 3-4 weeks resulting in a larger dose of radiation given daily over a shorter period of time. Two (2) to four (4) randomized controlled trials have shown that whole breast irradiation delivered after lumpectomy decreases local recurrence rates by 50%-60%.

Prone Breast Radiation Therapy

Prone Breast Radiation Therapy is designed for treatments of the left or right breast, including whole breast, partial breast, and accelerated partial breast treatments. Prone breast radiation therapy is a concept that has been recently perfected to treat all stages of breast cancer. Several recent studies have shown that receiving radiation to the breast while lying in the prone, or face down position has many benefits for women who are candidates for this type of treatment. This approach, while obtaining the same quality results as treatments in the traditional supine position, where women lay flat on their back for the radiation treatment, significantly avoids the radiation exposure to adjacent internal organs like the heart and lungs. The heart is especially vulnerable to damage when the left breast is treated because the heart is located on the left side of the chest just beneath the breast. Also, respiratory motion is reduced in the prone position, helping to improve treatment accuracy. Consequently, the prone breast position is most often used when radiating left breast cancer, although it can be used for treatment in both left and right breasts. Before the development of the prone breast technique, women with larger breasts were placed on their backs in the traditional supine position to receive radiation. Gravity pulls the breasts close to the body, causing exposure to internal organs and making treatment less consistent because larger breasts may lay flat differently with each radiation session. With the prone position, we can ensure radiation is distributed evenly, consistently and accurately during each treatment.

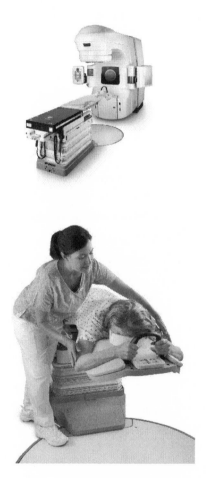

Advantages of Prone Breast Radiation Therapy:

- Radiation dose is evenly distributed in the breast
- Protects the heart and lungs from unwanted radiation
- Minimizes skin irritation
- Optimal cosmetic results

Below are examples of patients undergoing external beam radiation therapy in a modern linear accelerator using a dedicated prone breast treatment table device.

Advanced Breast Cancer

Technology has made it possible to be able to treat the entire chest wall and regional lymph nodes after receiving chemotherapy and surgery with minimal side-effects. In many cases, patients will be treated in the supine (lying on their backs) or prone (lying on their stomachs) positions. If a woman has more advanced or aggressive breast cancer, in many instances she might feel like giving up. This is mostly because of the lack of knowledge of what modern Radiation therapy can offer. If a woman has presented after many years of battling cancer with metastatic disease to the bones, brain or liver, there are techniques today that can focus and target only the tumor, using image guidance and avoiding normal structures (healthy tissue). This innovative technology is called Radiosurgery and it is usually delivered using a special piece of equipment specifically designed to destroy the tumor by using X-rays instead of surgery. The procedure is called Radiosurgery yet it is performed as an outpatient procedure without anesthesia or hospitalization. It is bloodless and painless and can be done in minutes, women should not be afraid to ask for this technology.

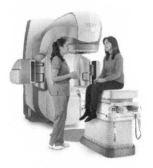

Radiosurgery: Stereotactic radiosurgery (SRS) uses numerous precisely focused radiation beams to treat tumors and other problems in the brain, neck and other parts of the body. It is not surgery in the traditional sense because there is no skin incision. Instead, SRS uses 3-D imaging to target high doses of radiation to the affected area with minimal impact on the surrounding healthy tissue. Like other forms of radiation, stereotactic radiosurgery works by damaging the DNA of the targeted cells. The affected cells then lose the ability to reproduce, which causes tumors to shrink. Stereotactic radiosurgery of the brain and spine is typically completed in a single session. Body radiosurgery is used to treat lung, liver, adrenal and other soft tissue tumors, and treatment typically involves multiple sessions, but no more than 5 sessions. When doctors use stereotactic radiosurgery to treat tumors in areas of the body other than the brain, it is usually called stereotactic body radiotherapy (SRBT) or stereotactic ablative radiotherapy (SABR).

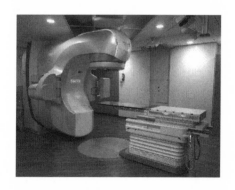

Brain Stereotactic Radiosurgery (SRS)

Brain metastases (BM) from breast cancer are associated with high morbidity and a poor prognosis. With Brain Stereotactic Radiosurgery (SRS), the tumor in the brain can be targeted directly with little to no radiation reaching the peripheral structures.

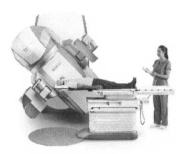

Extracranial Radiosurgery (Stereotactic Body Radiation Therapy) for Oligometastases

For women with advanced tumors, it is crucial that they are educated in all the new techniques and therapies available. Today, we are changing cancer from a fatal disease to a chronic disease that will require maintenance and follow-up, just like any other chronic illness. When Breast cancer becomes metastatic and has a few sites of disease (5 or less) it can be treated and is curable, this phase of cancer is known as oligometastatic disease. Stereotactic Body radiation Therapy (SBRT) is performed typically in 1 to 5 treatment sessions. Physicians directly supervise the treatments as is done in intracranial SRS. Typical treatment sessions for SBRT are longer than for conventional radiation therapy but because the treatment is finished in much fewer treatment sessions, the overall treatment time and resource utilization is considerably less than for conventional radiotherapy treatment.

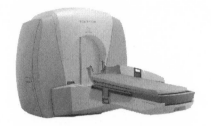

Spine Stereotactic Body Radiation Therapy (SBRT)

Spine SBRT has been used successfully as a palliative treatment for spine metastases either at first diagnosis or as a retreatment. Although this treatment modality is typically not offered in the setting of oligometastases, it can be considered as a standalone treatment for patients with limited bone metastases.

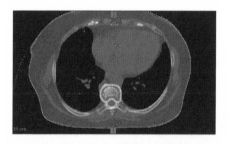

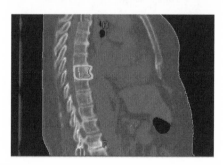

Liver and other systemic SBRT

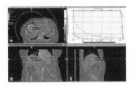 Reports of favorable clinical outcome after surgical resection of limited metastatic disease lend support to the investigation of SBRT as a noninvasive means of achieving the same goal; namely, eradication of recognized gross deposits of microscopic disease for the purpose of eliminating or greatly reducing the overall burden of systemic disease within the patient. SBRT has become popular for patients with a limited number of metastatic tumors to the liver [oligometastases = less than five (5)]. Even large lesions can be treated safely with modern dedicated radiotherapy units. Most studies show local control rates of higher than 70%.

~

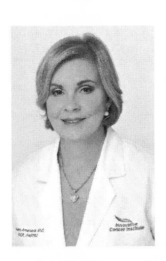

Beatriz E. Amendola, MD FACR FASTRO FACRO Fellow of the American College of Radiology (FACR), Fellow of the American Society of Radiation

Oncology 9 FASTRO) and Fellow of the American College of Radiation Oncology (FACRO)

Dr. Beatriz Amendola is a highly respected radiation oncologist and an honored member of the leading medical societies of the specialty in the United States, Latin America and Europe. She has been a highly successful practicing physician of radiation oncology in the U.S. for more than 35 years.

Dr. Beatriz Amendola completed her residency in Radiation Oncology at the Medical College of Virginia

in Richmond, VA., with Board Certification in Therapeutic Radiology by the American Board of Radiology in 1980. She has held several academic positions, including Acting Chairman of Department of Radiation Oncology at the University of Michigan and Associate Professor and Director of Residency Training at the University of Miami, Department of Radiation Oncology.

Dr. Beatriz Amendola has delivered more than 500 scientific presentations, scientific exhibits, and lectures nationally and internationally. She has received multiple honors and awards including the Gold Medal from CRILA (Circulo de Radioterapeutas Ibero Latino Americano). In 2015 Dr. Beatriz Amendola was awarded Honorary Membership in the Spanish Society of Radiation Oncology (SEOR) because of her multiple contributions to the specialty of Radiation Oncology in Spain. She has organized multiple educational courses and meetings on cancer treatment, specialty breast cancer, throughout Latin America.

Dr. Beatriz Amendola's Credentials and Previous Positions:

A Board certified in Therapeutic Radiology by the American Board of Radiology in 1980

Residency in Radiation Oncology completed at Medical College of Virginia, Richmond, VA

Associate Professor, Department of Radiation Oncology, University of Michigan, Ann Arbor, MI

Acting Chairman, Department of Radiation Oncology, University of Michigan

Director of Residency Training, Department of Radiation Oncology, Hahnemann University, Philadelphia, PA

Associate Professor, Director of Residency Training, University of Miami, Dept. of Radiation Oncology, Miami, FL

Clinical Associate Professor, Florida International University Herbert Wertheim School of Medicine, Miami, FL

Clinical Associate Professor, NOVA Southeastern University College of Osteopathic Medicine, Fort Lauderdale, FL

Founder and Director of Innovative Cancer Institute and the Brachytherapy Institute of South Florida

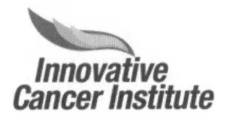

You can reach her at the Innovative Cancer Institute at (305) 669-6833 or via www.innovativecancer.com

6

PLASTIC SURGERY OPTIONS FOR BREAST CANCER RECONSTRUCTION

DEIRDRE MARSHALL, M.D., F.A.C.S AND ERIN WOLFE, B.S.

When a patient chooses to undergo breast reconstruction, she is faced with numerous treatment options to reconstruct the breast. Breast reconstruction is the rebuilding of a breast, utilizing prosthetic implants or one's own tissue to create a new breast with a natural appearance. Breast reconstruction not only restores the appearance of the breasts, it also leads to improved self-esteem and quality of life. Federal law mandates insurance coverage of breast reconstruction following mastectomy for breast cancer.

Surgical treatment of breast cancer includes partial removal of the breast (lumpectomy), and complete breast removal (mastectomy). Following lumpectomy, and sometimes mastectomy, patients may be treated with radiation therapy. In addition, patients may undergo pre-surgical and/or post-operative chemotherapy. Patients may choose to undergo breast reconstruction following removal of tissue for breast cancer.

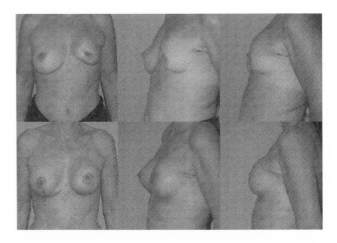

Figure 1. Breast reconstruction with implants following
lumpectomy and radiation

In cases where the tumor is multi-focal (in several areas of the breast), or a good cosmetic outcome is not possible with a lumpectomy, the patient may undergo reconstructive surgery to restore a normal appearance to the breast. Patients may alternatively choose to undergo a mastectomy, followed by breast reconstruction.

Nipple-sparing and skin-sparing mastectomies are an option if the tumor is distant from the nipple-areolar complex. This type of mastectomy may also be carried out in patients who do not have cancer, but who carry a breast cancer gene.

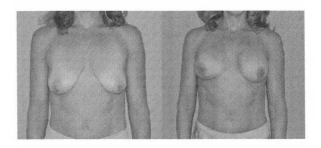

Figure 2. Skin sparing and nipple areolar sparing
mastectomies

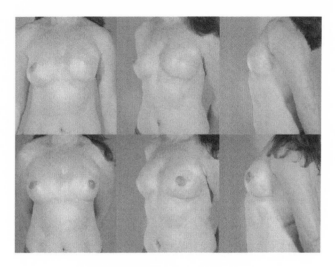

Figure 3. Nipple Areolar Reconstruction

Following mastectomy, breast reconstruction may be carried out at the time of mastectomy, or in a delayed fashion, depending on a variety of factors. Breast reconstruction utilizes implants and/or the patient's own tissues.

Implant-based breast reconstruction

Implant-based breast reconstruction is the most common technique used for breast reconstruction. Implant-based breast reconstruction may be performed immediately following mastectomy, or later, following the mastectomy procedure. In staged breast reconstruction, the surgeon inserts a tissue expander (a temporary implant) into the breast, underneath a pocket under the pectoralis major muscle of the chest wall. Acellular human or porcine dermal matrix may be used to completely wrap the implant, which allows the implant to be anchored in a stable position on the chest wall and increases soft-tissue coverage of the implant. This may improve the functional and cosmetic result. The use of dermal matrix grafts may minimize the development of post-operative implant capsular contraction (formation of tight scar tissue around the implant).

Following expander placement, saline solution is injected into the expander to increase its volume and to stretch the surrounding breast envelope. Subsequent surgery includes expander removal, permanent implant placement, and nipple-areolar reconstruction.

In direct to implant ("one-step") breast reconstruction, an implant is placed immediately following mastectomy, and expanders are not used. This approach can be used in patients who have generous and healthy soft tissue envelopes at the time of mastectomy. After a Direct-to-Implant breast reconstruction, patients may require a second operation to perfect breast contour, symmetry, size, and nipple-areolar aesthetics.

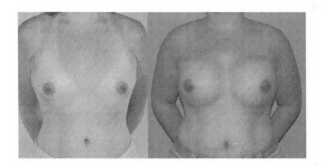

Figure 4. Bilateral prophylactic mastectomies and
Direct-to-Implant breast reconstruction

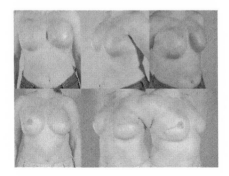

Figure 5. "Teardrop" anatomic shaped silicone gel
implants

Pre-pectoral breast reconstruction is the latest variant of direct implant breast reconstruction. In this procedure, the breast implant is placed on top of the pectoralis major muscle. This serves to decrease post-operative pain and decrease "animation deformity", which is the distortion of the breast implant caused by flexion of the chest wall muscles.

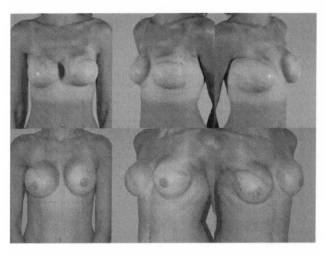

Figure 6. Revision: An improved aesthetic appearance can be as simple as implant exchange and tattooing

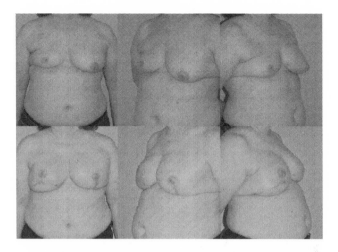

Figure 7. Revision following recurrent breast cancer:
An undesirable outcome, but a chance to achieve a
more even appearance of the breasts through revision

Autologous breast reconstruction

Autologous breast reconstruction, or "flap" reconstruction, is a surgical technique that uses the patient's own tissues to reconstruct the breast following mastectomy. Tissue is taken from a variety of donor sites that may include the abdomen, back, buttocks, or thighs. Breast reconstruction flaps may be either "pedicled" or "free." Pedicled flaps remain attached to the blood supply from the original donor site. Free flaps are removed completely from the body and are reattached to blood vessels in the region of the breast with microsurgical techniques. Flap reconstruction, using the patient's own tissues, is useful for patients who have had radiation, excessive scarring, or serious problems with implants.

1. Pedicled Flaps

i. TRAM flap: Transverse Rectus Abdominis Myocutaneous Flap

In a TRAM flap procedure, tissue from the abdomen is transferred, with its blood supply attached, to the mastectomy site.

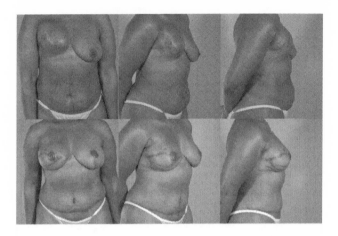

Figure 8. Unsatisfactory irradiated right breast implant
reconstruction converted to TRAM flap reconstruction

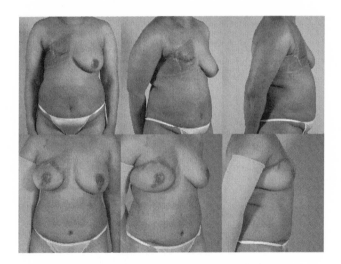

Figure 9. Delayed right breast reconstruction and
immediate left breast reconstruction with TRAM flaps.

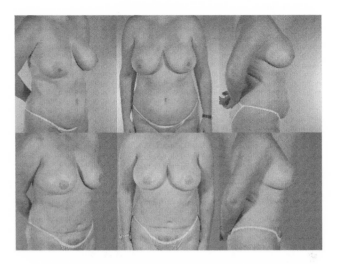

Figure 10. Immediate bilateral breast reconstruction
with TRAM Flaps

ii. Latisimuss Dorsi Myocutaneous (muscle and skin) Flap

The latissimus dorsi myocutaneous flap uses donor tissue from the back. A portion of the latissimus dorsi muscle gives blood supply to this flap without creating donor site dysfunction. This flap can be used to reconstruct small breasts without an implant, or it can also be used to increase the amount of soft-tissue coverage over an implant. This flap is very useful for patients who have had chest wall irradiation.

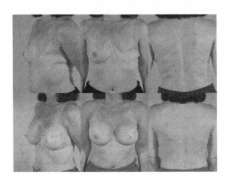

Figure 11. Left breast reconstruction with latissimus flap
and right breast augmentation

2. Free Flaps

i. Deep inferior epigastric perforator (DIEP) and superficial inferior epigastric artery (SIEP)

The DIEP and SIEA flaps are abdominal flaps that are used for breast reconstruction. These techniques are very similar, utilizing different donor site blood vessels.

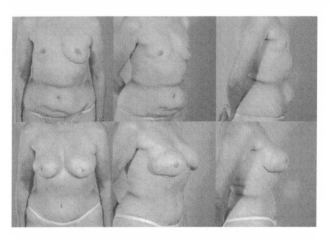

Figure 12. Double DIEP flap: Improve other areas of the body through breast reconstruction

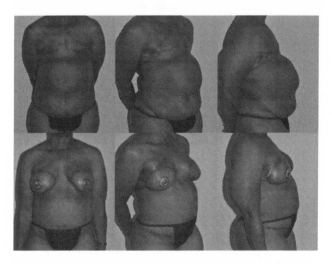

Figure 13. Double delayed bilateral breast reconstruction with DIEP Flaps

i. Superior and Inferior Gluteal Artery Perforator Flaps (IGAP, SGA)

The superior gluteal artery perforator flap (SGAP) and the inferior gluteal artery perforator flap (IGAP) are perforator flaps which utilize skin and fat from the buttocks.

Nipple-Areolar Reconstruction

When the nipple-areolar complex must be sacrificed in a mastectomy, the surgeon can employ a variety of techniques to reconstruct the nipple-areolar complex. These techniques employ a combination of rearrangement of local soft tissue, placement of full-thickness skin grafts, and tattooing with natural pigments.

Choosing the Best Option for Breast Reconstruction

When seeking breast reconstruction, a patient should select a board-certified plastic surgeon who has extensive experience in this field. Patients must understand that breast reconstruction is far more complex than cosmetic breast surgery. Often, breast reconstruction equates to making something out of nothing. Breast reconstruction is always carried out in stages. Even the best reconstruction result cannot re-create what mother nature can make.

References

1. https://www.ncbi.nlm.nih.gov/pmc/articles/PMC4717291/
2. https://www.ncbi.nlm.nih.gov/books/NBK470317/
3. https://www.ncbi.nlm.nih.gov/pmc/articles/PMC4717291/
4. https://www.ncbi.nlm.nih.gov/pubmed/15943735
5. https://www.ncbi.nlm.nih.gov/pubmed/21617423
6. https://www.ncbi.nlm.nih.gov/pubmed/29064917
7. https://www.ncbi.nlm.nih.gov/pubmed/27988412

8. https://www.ncbi.nlm.nih.gov/pmc/articles/PMC2884724/
9. https://www.ncbi.nlm.nih.gov/pubmed/24281592
10. https://www.ncbi.nlm.nih.gov/pubmed/16862569
11. https://www.ncbi.nlm.nih.gov/pubmed/22395342
12. https://www.ncbi.nlm.nih.gov/pmc/articles/PMC3255143/
13. https://www.ncbi.nlm.nih.gov/pubmed/18677130
14. https://www.ncbi.nlm.nih.gov/pubmed/20574484
15. https://www.ncbi.nlm.nih.gov/pubmed/2256348
16. https://www.ncbi.nlm.nih.gov/pubmed/21200195
17. https://www.ncbi.nlm.nih.gov/pubmed/19083539
18. https://www.ncbi.nlm.nih.gov/pubmed/25289266
19. https://www.ncbi.nlm.nih.gov/pubmed/11007387

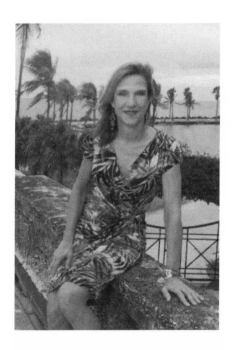

Deirdre Marshall, M.D., F.A.C.S. is a board certified plastic surgeon in Miami, and one of Florida's leading physicians in the plastic surgery specialty. For the last 20 years, she has held medical licenses in four states, as well as two board certifications in plastic and reconstructive surgery. In 2009, Dr. Marshall was named to South Florida's "Super Doctors" list. Additionally, she is considered an expert breast reconstruction and pediatric cranial, facial and hand surgeon. Dr. Marshall has taken several overseas surgical missions to Vietnam and various locations in Central and South America to educate and provide treatment to children in indigent and poverty-stricken areas.

Dr. Marshall graduated from Yale University. She completed her medical degree at the Stanford School of Medicine in Palo Alto, California, where she completed internship and residency in a combined program in general surgery and plastic and reconstructive surgery. Dr. Marshall has also completed fellowship training in hand and microsurgery in Paris and cosmetic surgery in Miami Beach. A highly respected plastic surgeon in Miami, Dr. Marshall has been honored with numerous academic awards and honors, including the Katherine M. McCormick Foundation Award for Women in Medicine and the Stanford University School of Medicine Research Honors Award.

Erin Wolfe, B.S., University of Miami Miller School of Medicine co-authored this chapter.

7

AUTOLOGOUS BREAST RECONSTRUCTION WITH EXTERNAL EXPANSION AND FAT GRAFTING

ROGER KHOURI M.D., RICHARD NADAL M.D., AND DANIEL CALVA, M.D.

Percutaneous Autologous Breast Reconstruction
External Vacuum Expansion and Autologous Fat Transfer
(EVE + AFT)
"Fat grafting breast reconstruction using small holes with percutaneous methods is an extremely versatile departure from the traditional approach to breast reconstruction allowing a more precise method of molding the tissues while at the same time providing the flexibility to enhance specific areas of the breast."

Key Learning Points

- Autologous breast reconstruction with AFT and EVE is safe
- There are no risks of cancer recurrence with EVE and AFT
- There are no issues with surveillance of the reconstructed breast after EVE and AFT

- EVE and AFT is a safe and effective alternative to traditional autologous flap breast reconstruction
- EVE allows greater grafting ability, and increases the overall volume retention of the reconstructed breast

The field of medicine continues to evolve, and plastic surgery is no different. Plastic surgery takes its name from the Greek word "Plastikos" which means "capable of being shaped or molded." In this chapter, we will see how advances in technology and refinements in surgical instrumentation now allow plastic surgeons to perform true tissue molding in breast reconstruction through a series of minimally invasive outpatient procedures. We will describe our experience at the Miami Breast Center with Fat Grafting, also known as autologous fat transfer (AFT), in breast reconstruction. Our protocol pays special attention to preoperative preparation and postoperative care. Active patient participation before and after the surgery is key to a successful outcome, and can help decrease the number of procedures required.

Breast reconstruction is typically performed in stages. The objectives are: the creation of a breast mound, creation of a nipple-areola complex, and achieving optimal symmetry. For various reasons, we often have to manipulate the other breast with a reduction, lift, or augmentation in order to achieve proper symmetry. As we saw in that chapter, there are now many alternatives when it comes to reconstruction following any type of ablative surgery for breast cancer. There is no perfect technique and each has its advantages and disadvantages.

Why Fat?

Reconstruction of the breast mound requires the addition of volume to compensate for the volume of tissue removed. Fat is found throughout the body and can be removed from areas where it is not wanted and placed in areas where it is needed. It is harvested by low negative pressure liposuction, and injected into the breast in small volumes to create, or add volume to, the breast mound. To be successful, it is essential to respect the tissue requirements for graft survival. We accomplish this by observing meticulous technique during the harvesting, processing, and grafting procedure. With proper technique, large volume fat grafting can now be performed safely and effectively, exactly what breast reconstruction requires. Either by itself, or in combination with other procedures, fat grafting has now become a practical alternative in breast reconstruction. It also has the added benefit of improving the overall shape of the body in the areas from which the fat is taken.

History

While fat grafting to the breast has been tried since the late nineteenth century, it wasn't until the last decade that it became popularized throughout the world. The combination of mammography, breast ultrasound imaging, and MRIs make the screening and diagnosis of breast cancer more precise. Suspicious lesions can now be differentiated from artifacts, such as calcifications resulting from injected fat. Thus, major hurdles in the implementation of fat grafting have been addressed, and this procedure can now deliver consistent results with properly planned outpatient fat grafting sessions. It is now accepted as a viable alternative in breast surgery by major plastic surgery societies as a safe and effective procedure that does not increase the risk of cancer.

Theory of Fat Grafting, Tissue Molding and Percutaneous Surgery

Fat survival after grafting is essential if it is to be a reliable method of reconstruction. In other words, the grafted cells have to survive once they are placed in the recipient tissue. While normal tissue is usually quite ready to accept a modest amount of volume, previous surgery or radiation can create a more hostile environment for the survival of these delicate fat cells. The proposed recipient of the graft has to be prepared in order to provide an adequate bed much like the preparation and irrigation of arid land prior to planting a crop. This is where we need the patient's help. We utilize preoperative external vacuum expansion by applying a suction cup known as The EVE system, which we will discuss in more detail in the next section. Briefly, it applies a three dimensional pull on the tissues of the surface of the chest that allows the tissues to expand; increasing the size of the recipient and improving its blood supply. We can then graft more fat, and maximize the chance of survival by optimizing our conditions.

Even so, the surgeon then has to determine the correct amount of fat to be grafted in order to avoid over-grafting. If too much fat is grafted, the pressure in the tissue will rise, compromise the capillary blood supply, and the graft fails. We use dilute fat on purpose to allow fluid absorption after surgery. Tissue pressure decreases and fat survival improves. We also depend on the EVE system before surgery to help by stretching the tissues before surgery. The larger space can accept more volume than could otherwise be safely grafted. In this way we can decrease the number of procedures required in the creation of a breast mound.

As always, proper instrumentation is necessary for the success of any procedure by providing efficiency, precision and safety. Specialized instruments developed at The Miami Breast Center for fat harvesting and grafting increase efficiency by economy of movement. This facilitates the procedure and allows the required precision for optimal fat graft survival. By improving efficiency, the surgeon can also save precious time under anesthesia without compromising the consistency of the results.

Special instrumentation is also required to break up deep scars and permit movement and molding of the tissue. During the grafting process deep scars are released then injected with fat so as to separate portions of the scar itself. We call this changing the cicatrix into a matrix. After a few sessions the tissue becomes softer and its quality and mobility improves. It can then be properly molded by percutaneous suturing.

Percutaneous surgery refers to surgery that is performed through the skin via needle sticks rather than typical incisions. It is a minimally invasive way to manipulate the tissues without significant scarring. Liposuction is a type of percutaneous surgery. AFT is another type of intervention that relies on percutaneous surgery. For purposes of tissue shaping we have also developed special instrumentation that allows us to mold the tissues using different suturing techniques to advance tissues percutaneously. Recruiting tissue from the upper abdomen and the side of the chest percutaneously allows us build a breast mound without major surgery or the scarring associated with other techniques. For symmetry, we can also reduce, lift and/or augment the opposite side percutaneously. Percutaneous suturing is a powerful tool in harnessing the benefits of adjacent tissue recruitment into the breast mound with less morbidity than the more traditional flaps.

Preoperative Preparation and The EVE Protocol

Prior to AFT, a preoperative MRI is essential to evaluate the soft tissues under the mastectomy flaps, or the remaining breast gland if a partial mastectomy was performed. The MRI is a critical component not only to evaluate for any potential recurrence, but also for long term follow-up and evaluation for any potential complications. The MRI is performed with a contrast called Gadolinium, and patients are screened for any potential allergies to the contrast, for renal or liver insufficiency, and for pregnancy, which might preclude the use of the contrast. Gadolinium contrast is necessary in breast MRI since it improves the clarity of the scanned images and internal structures.

ℰxternal 𝒱acuum ℰxpander

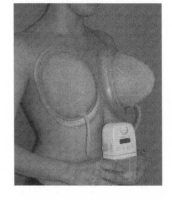

EVE

We take our time educating patients who are contemplating breast reconstruction with EVE assisted tissue expansion and AFT. It may take several educational sessions and emailed tutorials in order to familiarize patients on how to wear and cycle the EVE system. In the office, the patient will have a trial using the EVE device. This typically consists of a suction cycle over a 20 min period wearing the EVE device. The specific size of the EVE device will be selected depending on the patient's chest dimensions and breast size. The patient then decides if she can tolerate the cycles and wishes to proceed with EVE assisted tissue expansion and AFT.

EVE is started 2-3 weeks prior to surgery. The patients are instructed on how to apply and operate the device, and we monitor their progress during the preoperative period. Patients wear the EVE system for four hours the first day, adding two hours every day until they reach 14 hours per day of continuous wear. The EVE device is then utilized for 14 hours a day until the day of surgery, alternating pressures from 60-0-60 mmHg for 3-1-3 min. The recommended final total dose prior to AFT is 200 hours of breast expansion with the EVE system in the final two weeks prior to surgery.

When EVE is used correctly we expect to see some swelling,

superficial bruising, and blistering of the expanded skin as well as small red spots on the skin known as petechiae, which result from capillary rupture. These changes are temporary and resolve on their own after surgery. Their presence indicates that the soft tissues are well expanded and optimized for autologous fat grafting. Applying Opsite or Tegaderm on the skin can minimize blistering and helps prevent irritation.

We typically do not use EVE in patients that have implants. In this situation, the tissue simply pulls away from the implant and does not expand. Our approach is to downsize the implants and replace the implant volume with fat. The implants can eventually be removed altogether with the help of percutaneous suturing in one of the fat grafting sessions if that is the objective.

Each Patient is Different

Reconstruction with fat grafting can be performed in a complete mastectomy whether immediate or delayed, skin or nipple sparing. It has a role in reconstruction after breast conservation surgery with lumpectomy and radiation. It also gives us an additional tool as a "salvage" procedure when other techniques have failed. Fat grafting with percutaneous surgery is an extremely versatile departure from the traditional approach to breast reconstruction, allowing a more precise method of molding and shaping the tissues while at the same time providing the flexibility to enhance specific areas of the breast.

In the immediate reconstruction, the first stage is performed at the time of mastectomy. This is the perfect opportunity to add fat prior to the onset of scarring. It adds volume, minimizes the detrimental effects of postoperative scarring, and prepares the terrain for a greater volume of fat grafting in the next procedure. In many cases, immediate reconstruction with fat grafting can provide sufficient cleavage to simulate a social breast after the mastectomy. We can even perform what we call a delayed immediate reconstruction. This occurs when a patient has her mastectomy in her hometown and a few days later proceeds with fat grafting. If radiation therapy is planned postoperatively however, we prefer to preserve valuable fat until radiation has been completed.

In delayed primary reconstruction the first stage is performed several months or years after the mastectomy. The number of procedures depends on whether or not the patient has had radiation. Without radiation, breast mound reconstruction may be achieved in approximately three outpatient sessions. With radiation it may be up to six.

In breast conservation surgery a lumpectomy is followed by radiation therapy. This typically preserves much of the breast tissue depending on the original size of the breast. However, the remaining breast tissue has to be radiated in order to control local disease. Radiation will then lead to local tissue scarring that is difficult to contain and difficult to reconstruct. We have found that the best time to proceed with fat grafting is immediately after the end of radiation. The swelling in the tissues can provide safe sanctuary for a fat graft and the graft can help prevent many of the changes resulting from the radiation itself. We can take advantage of this adversary and turn it into an opportunity. It is quite a change from the traditional way of thinking.

Unfortunately, there are times when other reconstructive procedures fail. It is reassuring to know that fat grafting is still available as an option to complete the breast reconstruction. With patience and dedication, the scarred tissue in these very difficult cases can be slowly softened and augmented to the point where sufficient soft tissue molding is possible. It may take some extra procedures, but a very reasonable result can usually be obtained.

Revising a previously reconstructed breast can pose significant challenges depending on the existing situation. We carefully analyze the patient needs, the amount and quality of the tissues along with residual scarring, and establish realistic objectives.

Each situation requires an individually designed plan of action. Each series of procedures is specifically tailored to address the particular needs of the patient. From our perspective, each patient is different.

Postoperative Care and Follow-Up

The follow up period and care are ongoing, and patients are followed for life. The postoperative care includes prevention of fat re-absorption, identifying possible complications, and evaluating for the need of future surgical interventions. Before surgery, EVE expands the soft tissue in preparation for grafting. After surgery, the EVE expanded tissue has been turned from a cicatrix into a matrix occupied with small droplets of fat grafts. However, the healing process can create fibrosis and cause the expanded fat grafted matrix to contract. We like to maintain the matrix as large as possible to allow the maximum amount of fat to survive. Therefore, after the first week, the patient is encouraged to wear the EVE device as much as possible to maintain the matrix expanded. Once the fat survives, the fat graft will maintain the matrix expanded. This will allow a greater amount of fat to be grafted in a subsequent session.

Most planed re-interventions are done within a 3-6 month period. This allows the prior fat graft to stabilize, and the inflammatory process to subside. Only after the inflammation subsides, will the surgeon know the extent of graft survival. It is at this point that the patient and surgeon will have a more accurate understanding of how much volume or shaping is still needed. The particular goals of the next procedure can then be determined. A post-operative MRI is always performed 6 months following the last procedure.

Conclusion

Fat grafting has been found to have many beneficial effects on local tissue. By breaking up the scar tissue and introducing fat we can ultimately decrease the amount of contracture and improve the overall quality and mobility of the tissue. With percutaneous surgery the tissue can then be shaped as needed. The fat is used for volume enhancement and at the same time as a glue to hold the molded tissue in its new position.

Percutaneous surgery with AFT is a twenty first century procedure, a paradigm departure from the mutilating patch-like flap reconstruction, and from the insertion of foreign body implants. It empowers women with the ability to regenerate, in situ, beautiful and sensate breasts without incisions. The process takes time. Reconstructing a new breast requires patience and compliance with EVE use. At the Miami Breast Center we have developed a reliable intervention that optimizes the success of each fat grafting session thereby decreasing the number of procedures required. It has many advantages over traditional methods of reconstruction. It is performed in an outpatient setting, it has less morbidity and has been shown to lower costs. With this excellent alternative, we are at the forefront of breast reconstruction.

References

1. R.K. Khouri, J.M. Smit, E. Cardoso, et al. "Percutaneous aponeurotomy and lipofilling: A regenerative alternative to flap reconstruction?" *Plast Reconstr Surg.* 132.5 (2013): 1280–1290. Print.

2. R.K. Khouri, G. Rigotti, E. Cardoso, et al. "Megavolume Autologous Fat Transfer: Part I. Theory and Principles." *Plast Reconstr Surg.* 133.3 (2014): 550-557. Print.

3. R.K. Khouri, et al. "Megavolume Autologous Fat Transfer: Part II Practice and Techniques." *Plast Reconstr Surg.* 133.6 (2014): 1369-77. Print.

4. R.K. Khouri, G. Rigotti, et al. "Tissue-Engineered Breast Reconstruction with EVE-Assisted Fat Grafting: A 7-Year,

488-Patient, Multicenter Experience." *Plast Reconstr Surg.*
135.3 (2015): 643-658. Print.

~

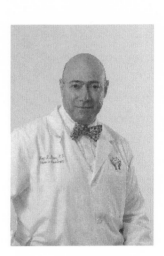

Roger Khouri, M.D., F.A.C.S is the founder of the Miami Breast Center. He has more than 30 years of experience as a reconstructive surgeon. He is the pioneer in breast reconstruction using external vacuum expansion and fat transfer. In 1999 he invented the BRAVA external expander, which led him to develop the now well-established and accepted third-option to breast reconstruction using percutaneous techniques for fat grafting to the breast. He recently developed the next generation breast external vacuum expansion device called EVE.

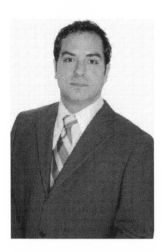

Daniel Calva-Cerqueira, M.D., F.A.C.S completed his training at the prestigious Johns Hopkins/University of Maryland Plastic & Reconstructive Surgery program. Straight out of training, he joined Dr. Khouri to learn the unique methods and techniques that are only performed at the Miami Breast Center. He has mastered his methods and helped advance and perfect these techniques.

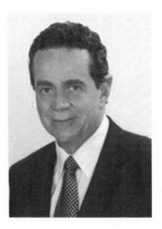

Richard D. Nadal, M.D., F.A.C.S., Board Certified in Plastic and Reconstructive Surgery. He earned his medical degree in 1979 and the University of Puerto Rico School of Medicine. He then continued his training in general surgery at the University of Florida and Washington

D.C. in Georgetown University. In 1985 he received his certification from the American Board of Surgery.

Dr. Nadal continued his training in plastic surgery at the Indiana University which included six months of neck and head surgery. He then continued his training and finished a fellowship at the prominent Manhattan Eye, Ear and Throat Hospital. In 1989 he was certified by the American Board of Plastic Surgery after completing a total of 8 years in the surgical training alongside the best in his field.

Afterwards he established himself in Miami, Florida where he continued practicing surgery for 18 years. He is an active member of the following organizations: American Society for Aesthetic Plastic Surgery, American Society of Plastic Surgeons, Fellow of the American College of Surgeons and Colegio de Médicos-Cirujanos de Puerto Rico.

Learn more about Dr. Nadal at www.miamibreastcenter.com.

8

SCAR WARS: SCAR REHABILITATION AFTER BREAST CANCER

JILL WAIBEL, M.D.

Healing after breast cancer can be an emotional, spiritual and physical journey for women. Physical healing often helps emotional healing. One powerful step in healing after breast cancer diagnosis and treatment is a successful reconstruction. A final part of reconstruction is the treatment of any scars created by either surgery.

IN THE BEGINNING

Scars are an unavoidable result of any surgery. The first step to achieving a minimal scar is optimal surgery and post-operative surgical care. It is imperative to follow the directions of the surgeons during the healing process. In the early days after surgery, you will be exhausted; the sutures in the wounds will not be pretty. But from the moment of surgery, you can start to decrease the potential for scars. A scar forms after surgery because your body produces collagen to fill in the injury made by surgery. Due to its location, the chest area can be a bit challenging because many incisions are under tension. In some cases, a body will overproduce collagen causing a red, thick scar called a hypertrophic scar. In other instances, the body will underproduce collagen and you may end up with an indented (atrophic) scar. Since a scar starts the moment of surgery, a great surgeon, meticulous post-operative care, and a laser dermatologist will help you along your path.

Breasts are an important part of a female and her identity. Being diagnosed with cancer can be devastating, not just physically, but emotionally. A scar often forces the patient to relive the diagnosis, fear, and treatment every time they undress.

After breast cancer, scars often become noticeable 1-6 months after surgery. Recovery after significant injury involves the coordinated restoration of form and function to maximize patient outcomes. Reconstructive efforts may be limited by the development and persistence of pathologic scar formation. Scars are areas of fibrous tissue that replace normal skin after injury. Scar tissue is of inferior functional & aesthetic quality to the tissue it replaces.

However, patients no longer have to live with the scars as there are now many treatment options to minimize the scars, improve how they look and feel, and control symptoms of itching and pain. In this chapter we will share scientific innovations and technologies currently in use and those being developed to help minimize scars.

Early Post-Operative Care

Once the sutures are removed or dissolve, which is typically about 10-14 days after surgery, we recommend compression using silicone sheets. Compression is very important because it tells the fibroblasts (cells that can make too much collagen) to calm down (1). In the lab, the compression turns off these cells and tells the skin to heal. Compression is most useful in preventing an elevated (or hypertrophic) scar. I usually tell patients to use compression that they find comfortable 24/7 for the first six months. By the seventh month after surgery, most scars won't grow much more so it is usually fine to stop compression unless a complex scar has developed, then defer to your scar specialist to guide you. Next find the nearest laser expert!

Under Construction: Treatment Options for Scars After Breast Cancer

Scars are the result of wounds that affect millions of people in the world. The initial injury may be caused by surgery. Despite the best surgical care, patients continue to have functional impairments and uncomfortable symptoms from scars. Severe cutaneous scars are disfiguring and have many associated symptomatology including pruritus, pain, decreased function and restricted range of motion (2). The new goal for scar treatment is that definitive reconstruction ends with recovery of optimal appearance and function.

Scarring following trauma and reconstructive surgery is difficult to predict, and both patients and physicians are focused on minimizing scar appearance. Preventative and passive treatment options include pressure therapy, silicone therapies, and massage.

Several non-operative modalities are available to improve hypertrophic scars. Intralesional injections of anti-inflammatory and antimitotic agents have been widely used to decrease scar thickness and they often decrease itching (3). A series of treatments one month apart are often necessary for the desired effect and are also used in combination with other therapies. Agents commonly used include triamcinolone acetonide and 5-fluorouracil (5-FU). The mechanism of action is to reduce fibroblast proliferation and can lead to improvement in hypertrophic scarring. Typically, these agents are used in combination with lasers and operative modalities for synergistic improvement in outcomes.

Let There Be Light: Laser Therapy to Improve Breast Scars

The ability to remodel a scarred dermis and epidermis via laser therapy yield results not previously possible until the past decade with the invention of fractional lasers. A fractional laser is not only a box of light, but also a box of hope. A photon is a particle of light – ordinary white light comes from spontaneous emissions of photons.

Lasers is an acronym which stands for Light Amplification by Stimulated Emission of Radiation. Lasers use light to heal. A laser is a powerful tool to deal with scar complications & deformities.

Multiple therapeutic options have been used to improve scars. When reepithelization of skin and the best surgery have taken their course, there are now new laser options for further scar improvements in function, symptoms and cosmesis. Lasers are a scientifically precise and effective treatment modality to rehabilitate and improve scars (4). Lasers have added a powerful tool to improve scar symptoms and deformities.

THE HUMAN BODY CAN HEAL THE SMALLEST WOUND EVER ENCOUNTERED (FRACTIONAL WOUND) IN SCAR TISSUE & THE HEALING RESULTS IN (ALMOST) NORMAL SKIN

It has been well studied that gentle, early laser intervention can treat a scar and prevent further scarring. Many patients and surgeons think that you should wait a year before laser, but it is quite the opposite – scars are more pliable and can be stopped with early laser intervention (5).

SCAR LASER PHYSICS

We do not fully understand the biological basis by which scars improve after laser therapy. Scarring is a tissue response, acquired during the second trimester of fetal development at the same time of cellular immunity (6). In fact, infants inside the uterus up to the second trimester don't scar. We are still trying to harness this special environment and bring this to adults but so far have not succeeded. Scar tissue has increased vascular and lymphatic channels as well as changes in collagen structure compared to normal skin. However, in scars the blood vessels, lymphatics and collagen often are in a chaotic array with resultant decreased physiological function. It is known that in the treatment of healthy skin fractional ablative laser these microscopic thermal injuries are produced in the dermis which stimulate a wound healing cascade that ultimately leads to tissue remodeling (7). Normal skin can remodel these microscopic wounds without scarring. Macroscopic thermal burn injury causes the worst scars seen in clinical medicine. It is not understood how macroscopic thermal injury causes scars and microscopic thermal injury improves scars. The improvements appear to be in the epidermis and dermis, with effects in the adnexal skin structures. Many patients report immediate improvement in pruritus, pain and increased range of motion within hours to weeks after even one treatment session. The skin heals first with improvement of dyschromia followed in time with improvements in texture and topography.

DIFFERENT TYPES OF BREAST SCARS

Hypertrophic

Appearance: these scars are usually red, raised over surgical scar area – common after lumpectomy, mastectomy and / or reconstruction. They may fade with time but most will need treatment for optimal results (8).

Atrophic

Appearance: sunken, often white and can be caused when scars pull apart because a significant amount of tissue was removed or perhaps there was an infection after surgery (Figure 1). Treatment includes surgical revision, laser or laser assisted delivery with a biostimulator (9).

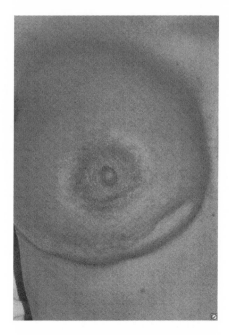

Figure 1a: 43-year-old Hispanic female with Fitzpatrick skin type IV with erythematous, hyperpigmented, atrophic scar.

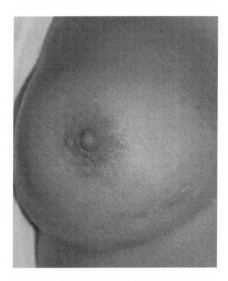

Figure 1b: Same patient after a total of 1 injectable treatments using a biostimulator.

Keloid

Appearance: scars tend to be reddish or purple in color, and often very large and ropey and have grown even beyond surgery area (Figure 2). These often run in the family and if a patient has a personal history of keloids, I like to do a pre-surgery prevent keloid plan and regular follow up appointments working with the surgeon's post-surgery (10).

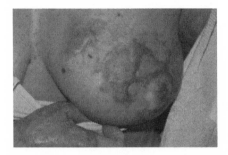

Figure 2a: 48-year-old Caucasian female with Fitzpatrick skin type III with erythematous, hyperpigmented, hypertrophic, keloid scar.

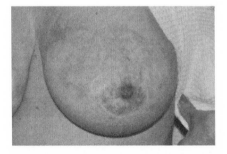

Figure 2b: Same patient after a total of 7 laser treatments using a multimodal approach with laser.

LASER & SURGERY SYNERGY FOR TREATMENT OF SCARS

If you develop or have developed a complex scar – don't worry! Your laser dermatologist and surgeon can work together to do scar revision. The treatment of scars is a multispecialty (different doctors from different specialties) endeavor (11). A combination approach with medical experts yield optimal scar improvements. If an injury heals in the presence of tension, hypertrophy often ensues. Understanding the role of tension in the development of a scar is essential to design a successful treatment strategy. If there is significant hypertrophy or contracture present in a scar, surgical intervention is necessary to relieve the tension or there is a high likelihood the scar with reform. After tension relief, hypertrophic and contracture scars are more elastic with new remodeling of collagen and are more amenable to treatment with laser (12). However, if a scar has had initial fractional laser therapy this often makes surgical intervention easier to perform due to thinner collagen bundles.

APPROACH TO TREATMENT OF CUTANEOUS SCARS

In the initial evaluation of the scar, the physician should determine what characteristics the scar possesses and then chose therapies to address these issues. Some factors to consider before choosing parameters of laser device include the thickness of scar (thicker scars need increased depth), age of scar (younger scars decrease depth and density), body location of the scar (off face decrease depth and density), skin type of the patient (darker skin types decrease density) and comorbid medical conditions (13). Next, determine if a scar is hypertrophic, keloid, contracture or atrophic. The dyschromia of a scar should be evaluated for erythema, hyperpigmentation and hypopigmentation. Often severe scars have multiple of these characteristics within the same scar. Our approach is to first use non-ablative laser to treat vascular & pigmented components of scar then to use fractional ablative devices for ablation of scar tissue, coagulation of microvasculature & stimulate subsequent neocollagenesis. The fractional ablative devices are the mainstay of therapy due to their ability to improve all scar types. Repeated laser sessions can occur until patient and/or physician satisfied. It is our clinical experience as well as published articles that with each laser session scars continue to improve with each laser session (14).

Surgical Scars

All surgical scars improve with fractional ablative laser (Figure 3-5). First, one must evaluate if the surgical scar is elevated (hypertrophic) or depressed (atrophic). The thicker hypertrophic scars need deeper treatment depths whereas more atrophic scars can be treated more superficially. Early surgical scars with significant erythema respond to vascular lasers with or without same day treatment of fractional lasers. In a study of 23 Korean women with thyroidectomy scars single session of 2 passes with a fractional CO_2 laser with a pulse energy of 50mJ, density of 100 spots/cm2. Treatments performed 2-3 weeks after surgery (15).

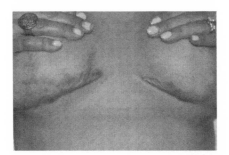

Figure 3a: 32-year-old Hispanic female with Fitzpatrick skin type IV with erythematous, hyperpigmented, hypertrophic surgical scar.

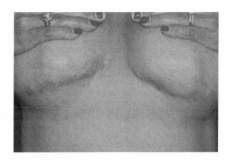

Figure 3b: Same patient after a total of 5 laser treatments
using a multimodal approach with lasers.

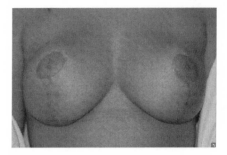

Figure 4a: 17-year-old Hispanic female with Fitzpatrick
skin type IV with erythematous, hyperpigmented
hypertrophic surgical scar.

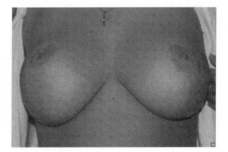

Figure 4b: Same patient after a total of 5 laser treatments
using a multimodal approach with lasers.

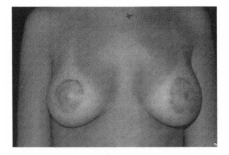

Figure 5a: 23-year-old Hispanic female with Fitzpatrick skin type IV with erythematous, hyperpigmented surgical scar.

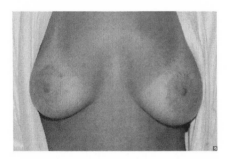

Figure 5b: Same patient after a total of 9 laser treatments using a multimodal approach with lasers.

Fractional Laser Treatment Technique

Most treatments are performed in the clinic setting using commercially available topical anesthetic preparations under occlusion for one hour or more prior to treatment. We also offer oral pain and anxiety pills and laughing gas to keep patients comfortable. You have suffered enough!

With previous discussion in mind, fractional laser treatment technique, parameters, and adjunctive treatments should be applied thoughtfully to minimize the degree of cumulative thermal injury to the tissue. Each treatment is customized at every session according to individual scar characteristics and interval changes. Selected pulse energies are proportional to the scar thickness as estimated by palpation and desired treatment depth without extending beyond the depth of the scar. Low-density fractional treatment is favored to reduce the risk of complications when treating scars. The treatment area includes the entire scar sheet and a one to two-millimeter rim of normal skin. Any part of the body may potentially be treated with fractional laser therapy.

When to Treat a Scar: Catch Scars Early!

The optimal time to begin fractional laser treatment has yet to be determined. As a rule, there should be a healed and intact epidermis prior to laser treatment. Younger, less mature scars are less tolerant of aggressive treatment and should be treated more judiciously in terms of laser settings and combination treatments than more mature scars (years after injury). Mature scars whether one-year-old or sixty-years-old all respond well to laser therapy. A minimum treatment interval of one to three months between fractional laser treatments is recommended to give scar tissue which is compromised time to heal. Even after just one treatment session a patient may continue to have improvement for many months up to one year.

Post-Operative Considerations

Immediately after ablative fractional treatments, petrolatum or a petrolatum-based ointment is applied and continued several times daily until the site is fully epithelialized, usually within three or four days. Cold compresses are helpful in first forty hours to decrease excessive edema and for patient comfort. Patients may resume showering and exercise the following day and begin gentle daily cleansing with mild soap of the area at least twice a day. Dilute vinegar compresses may be initiated according to the preference of the treating surgeon and patient preference. Vinegar may help pH of the skin return to more normal and promote healing as well as discourage bacterial or fungal colonization during this healing period. Patients are allowed to resume essentially normal activity after treatment. Sun avoidance is recommended for twelve weeks after laser therapy. In cases of scar contracture, participation in physical and occupational therapy is highly recommended to take full advantage of the laser effects. Full immersion such as in a pool or the ocean is not recommended until the treatment area is fully epithelialized to avoid infections. As with any cutaneous surgical procedure, basic contact and hygiene precautions should be emphasized. Oral antibiotics and antivirals are commonly used for prophylaxis starting one day prior to treatment and continuing up to one-week post laser treatment. Antifungals may be entertained on a case-by-case basis or if the patient develops localized pain or pruritus after laser treatment. Sun-protection should be advocated, including avoidance in the early post-treatment period and application of bland sun-protection once epithelial integrity is restored. Physical sun-protection of zinc or titanium dioxide are less irritating to newly lased skin. Compression therapy while healing from laser with either silicone gel sheets, tight athletic wear or medical compression garments. We recommend starting compression forty-eight hours after laser therapy.

Complications

Overall fractional ablative lasers have a favorable adverse event rate. Safe treatment is based on the avoidance excessive thermal injury and good laser practices in clinic. It is recommended if possible to see a patient one week after therapy to ensure skin has re-epithelization and no infections. Patients are advised to call if they experience excessive pain or pruritus.

Laser-Assisted Delivery of Drugs to Maximize Each Scar Treatment

Fractional laser technology has revolutionized scar laser therapy (16). The fractional ablative tunnels can be utilized for laser assisted delivery systems (LADS) of a variety of drugs, topical agents and other living tissue. Laser assisted drug delivery allows for greater precise depth of penetration by existing topical medications, more efficient transcutaneous delivery of large drug molecules, and even systemic drug administration via a transcutaneous route (Figure 5). These zones may be used immediately post-operatively to deliver drugs and other substances to synergistically create an enhanced therapeutic response.

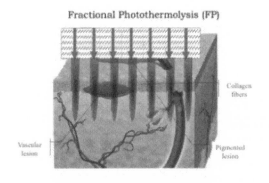

Figure 5: This photo demonstrates the channels created with a fractional ablative laser to allow greater depth of penetration of medications or cosmeceuticals.

Summary

Since their introduction, fractional lasers have helped many breast cancer survivors with scars. It is very rewarding to be a physician who is part of improving a scar on a woman cancer survivor. The patients and families are grateful for these medical devices. After the scar is treated and all are happy, we usually refer the patients onto nipple reconstruction, either building or tattooing.

I am always struck by the beautiful spirit, strength of character, and clarity of mind that cancer survivors gracefully acquire, and the way they truly appreciate life. The way breast cancer survivors live their lives, appreciate what is important, and rally for success in the face of life's greatest adversity, is an incredible daily source of inspiration. The medical success of lasers has added greatly to our ability to help heal our patients.

References

1. Minaev SV, Ivchenko AA, Babich II, Gerasimenko IN, Isaeva AV, Ivchenko GS, Kachanov AV, Bolotov YN. A new approach in the compression therapy of post-operative scars. *Khirurgiia (Mosk).* 2018;(2):79-84.

2. Xiao Y, Sun Y, Zhu B, Wang K, Liang P, Liu W, Fu J, Zheng S, Xiao S, Xia Z. Risk factors for hypertrophic burn scar pain, pruritus, and paresthesia development. *Wound Repair Regen.* 2018 May 2.

3. Waibel J, Wulkan AJ, Shumaker PR. Treatment of hypertrophic scars using laser and laser assisted corticosteroid delivery. *Lasers Surg Med.* 2013 Mar;45(3):135-40.

4. Issler-Fisher AC, Waibel JS, Donelan MD. Laser modulation of hypertrophic scars: technique and practice. *Clin Plast Surg.* 2017 Oct;44(4):757-766.

5. Karmisholt KE, Haerskjold A, Karilsmark T, Waibel J, Paasch U, Haedersdal M. Early intervention to reduce scar formation – a systemic review. *J Eur Acad Dermatol Venereol.* 2018 Feb 8.

6. Larson BJ, Longaker MT, Lorenz HP. Scarless fetal wound

healing: a basic science review. *Plast Reconstr Surg.* 2010 Oct;126(4): 1172-80.

7. Anderson RR, Parrish JA. Selective photothermolysis: precise microsurgery by selective absorption of pulsed radiation. *Science.* 1983 Apr 29;220(4596):524-7.

8. Gold MH, McGuire M, Mustoe TA, Pusic A, Sachdev M, Waibel J, Murcia C; International Advisory Panel on Scar Management. Updated international clinical recommendations on scar management: part 2 – algorithms for scar prevention and treatment. *Dermatol Surg.* 2014 Aug;40(8):825-31.

9. Rkein A, Ozog D, Waibel JS. Treatment of strophic scars with fractionated CO_2 laser facilitating delivery of topically applied poly-L-lactic acid. *Dermatol Surg.* 2014 Jun;40(6):624-31.

10. Zhao YX, Ho CK, Xie Y, Chen YH, Li HZ, Zhang GY, Li QF. Calcimycin suppresses S100A4 expression and inhibits the stimulatory effect of transforming growth factor βi on keloid fibroblasts. *Ann Plast Surg.* 2018 May 24.

11. Grimaldo A, Marziano C, Barone D, Bistolfi F. Multimodal treatment of locally advanced carcinoma of the breast. Experience at the galliera di Genova hospital. *Radiol Med.* 1990 Oct;80(4):514-8.

12. Monstrey S, Middelkoop E, Vranckx JJ, Bassetto F, Ziegler UE, Meaume S, Teot L. Updated scar management practical guidelines: non-invasive and invasive measures. *J Plast Reconstr Aesthet Surg.* 2014 Aug;67(8): 1017-25.

13. Zhou S, Cai J, Niu F, Zong X, Xu J, Du L, Chen G. Comparison of biological characteristics and quantity of epidermal stem cells from hypertrophic scar skin and normal skin of human beings. *Zhonghua Yi Xue Za Zhi.* 2014 Apr 15;94(14):1097-100.

14. AlGhamdi K, Khurrum H. Successful treatment of

atrophic facial leishmaniasis scars by CO_2 fractional laser. *J Cutan Med Surg.* 2014 Nov; 18(6):379-84.

15. Jung JY, Jeong JJ, Roh HJ, Cho SH, Chung KY, Lee WJ, Nam KH, Chung WY, Lee JH. Early postoperative treatment of thyroidectomy scars using a fractional carbon dioxide laser. *Dermatol Surg.* 2011 Feb;37(2):217-23.

16. Sklar LR, Burnett CT, Waibel JS, Moy RL, Ozog DM. Laser assisted drug delivery: a review of an evolving technology. *Lasers Surg Med.* 2014 Apr;46(4):249-62.

~

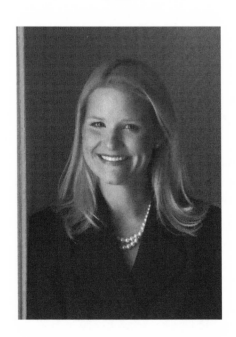

Jill S. Waibel, M.D. practices as a Board-Certified Dermatologist specializing in general dermatology, cutaneous laser surgery and cosmetic dermatology for adults and children. She is in private practice in Miami, Florida and Coral Gables, Florida. She is currently the Medical Director and Owner of the Miami Dermatology and Laser Institute in

Miami. Dr. Waibel is the Subsection Chief of Dermatology at Baptist Hospital.

In addition, Dr. Waibel serves as a Clinical Voluntary Assistant Professor at the University of Miami. She is a world-recognized leader in dermatologic laser surgery and lectures all over the world to train other physicians. In her practice she has over 65 laser devices and treats a wide variety of cutaneous disease. Dr. Waibel is active in basic science clinical trials at the University of Miami and has a clinical trials division Miami Dermatology and Research.

One of Dr. Waibel's primary passions is the treatment of scars by applying today's latest cutaneous laser technologies. She has success-fully developed industry-leading procedures and techniques with lasers, received numerous awards for her contributions to medicine, and published numerous peer-reviewed journal articles and several textbook chapters.

She was named "Person of the Week" on ABC World News Tonight in 2015 and was recently granted a Cutting Edge Research Grant by the American Society for Dermatologic Surgery. She has received numerous awards for her contributions to medicine, including an award given by Surgeon General Koop. The 2016 JDD Humanitarian Award has been given to Dr. Waibel for her innovative work in using lasers to treat patients with traumatic burn injuries. Dr. Waibel was also recently awarded the 2017 ASLMS Leadership, Mentorship & Public Advocacy for Women in Medical Science Award. Dr. Waibel lectures, collaborates and trains mili-tary physicians to help wounded warriors. She makes her home in Coral Gables with her husband and four children.

She can be reached via her office phone at (305) 279-6060, cell phone at (561) 313-1457, or by email at jwaibelmd@miamidermlaser.com.

9
POST-MASTECTOMY NIPPLE AREOLA TATTOOS

SUZANNE MOE

Following mastectomy and breast reconstruction, many women are left without a nipple or surrounding areola. For those who would like to complete their reconstruction by restoring the natural appearance of their nipple-areola complex, yet would prefer to avoid undergoing additional surgeries, there is a non-invasive, non-surgical option. Paramedical Micropigmentation, also known as paramedical tattooing, is an art form that helps to restore and softly redefine features that have been compromised or lost. It is a relatively easy procedure which involves depositing pigmented ink just below the epidermis (the outermost layer of skin) into the dermal layer of the skin (the layer of cells beneath the epidermis).

As a paramedical tattoo artist, I'm able to support the work of reconstructive plastic surgeons by replicating the natural color and shape of a nipple/areola with custom-mixed pigments that resemble natural skin tones. Realistic looking nipple areola tattoos can be created on women who have undergone bilateral or unilateral mastectomy, with or without nipple reconstruction. A new nipple areola can be matched to the existing native breast with a mix of various colors and shades to get the correct pigment. If there is no nipple, a nipple can be created artistically with light and shadow techniques, to give the illusion of depth and dimension. This is also known as a 3d nipple areola tattoo. These special tattoos provide the finishing touch to breast reconstruction and can help women feel better about themselves after a long journey. A common side effect is a renewed sense of self-confidence, a greater sense of wellbeing, and even a little giddiness and joy!

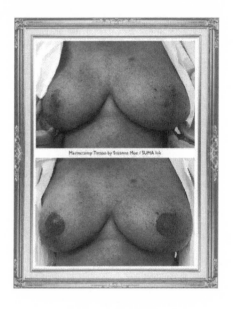

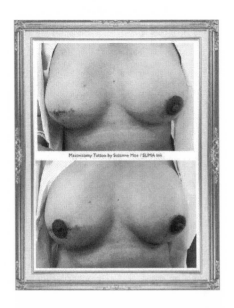

Mastectomy Tattoo by Suzanne Moe / SUMA Ink

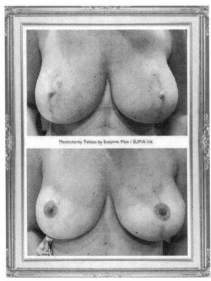

Mastectomy Tattoo by Suzanne Moe / SUMA Ink

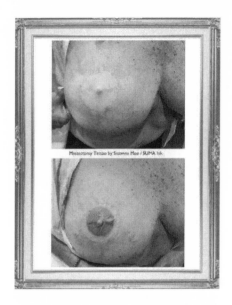

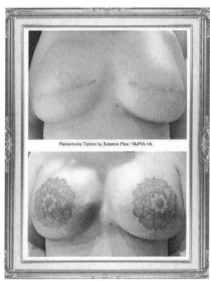

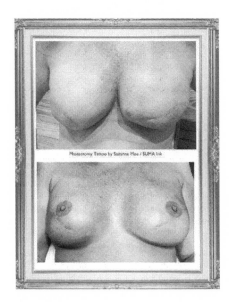

Mastectomy Tattoo by Suzanne Mae / SUMA Ink

It's important for women to feel empowered with a sense of control over how they would like their restored nipple-areola complex to look. If we were to work together, we would collaborate as a team. You could be both the canvas and the art director and I would work as your artist and technician. I'd also be happy to work together with your reconstructive surgeon to respectfully complete his/her work with the best possible outcome for all involved.

Below are some frequently asked questions:

How does the process generally work?

A consultation would be required prior to receiving your tattoo. This could take place in-person at the studio, or you could choose to have a "digital" consultation over the phone/internet. You would receive a medical health history form to fill out and tattoo care instructions to study. Three photos would be required: one photo of both breasts from the front, one close-up/left, one close-up/right. After I receive and review your health history and photos, we would talk about your design and color preferences. You would have the opportunity to ask any questions you might have. Your aftercare instructions would be reviewed and we would discuss your recommended service plan.

On the day of your service, the color, size, shape and placement will be confirmed and your custom ink colors mixed. An outline will be drawn around the area to be tattooed. Relaxing music will play in the background as you receive your tattoo. Very little discomfort is experienced during the procedure. Afterwards, your tattoo will appear brighter and darker than the actual ink used. Some swelling is normal. Your tattoo will be cleaned and covered with non-stick gauze. It's okay to wear a bra, as it can help hold the gauze in place.

The following 10-14 days will be dedicated to aftercare. The aftercare process is simple, but very important. You must keep the site clean, apply a healing ointment twice a day, and avoid direct sunlight, swimming and soaking in water during the first two weeks of receiving your new tattoo.

After 6 weeks, we'll evaluate your tattoo and determine if it needs additional color or not. It's much easier to tattoo darker pigment on a lighter canvas than the other way around, so I choose to tattoo conservatively, on the lighter side. If a second session is desired, that can be scheduled for 8-10 weeks after your first tattoo session.

Does it hurt?

The post-mastectomy reconstructed breast doesn't have the same sensation as it did before surgery, so tattooing the area is not usually painful. Pain tolerances differ however, depending on the individual and the type of breast reconstruction. Medical grade numbing cream can be used to ensure your comfort, if needed. The tattoo can feel a bit like a minor sunburn for a few days.

How long after my reconstructive surgery should I wait before I can get nipple areola tattoos?

It's important to give your body enough time for the sutures to completely dissolve, scars to mature and for the reconstructed breast to settle before receiving a tattoo. The tattoo should be the final step of your breast reconstruction journey, the finishing touch. With that being said, it's ideal to wait at least 6 months after reconstructive surgery (especially if there is direct scar involvement) with an absolute minimum of 4 months.

How long does an average tattoo session take?

The average length of time for a (bilateral) 3d nipple areola tattoo session is 2-1/2- 3 hours. This time includes paperwork, consultation, numbing time if required, the actual tattooing and breaks, if desired. The exact time, of course, varies with each individual.

What is the healing period like?

You should be able to return to work or your other daily activities immediately following the procedure without any embarrassment or discomfort. Moderate, mindful exercise is fine. Your tattoo will be a bit moist for the first few days, as ink, plasma and lymphatic fluid are excreted through the epidermis while healing.

You will keep your tattoo clean by washing it at least once a day with an unscented antibacterial soap and applying a thin film of healing ointment on it for 10-14 days. During this period, you will notice the color soften into your skin and look more and more natural.

In approximately 3-7 days after your tattoo service, the top layer of skin will begin to exfoliate (quite like a reptile shedding its skin) and a new layer of skin will regenerate. The cells within this new layer of skin will be void of pigment, so your tattoo will appear lighter and more translucent as it heals. This process takes about a week and may be a bit itchy. Refrain from scratching or picking the tattoo site during this time to ensure proper pigment retention and optimal healing.

Is nipple areola tattooing safe?

I utilize a 100% single-use, disposable system for each procedure and my methods of tattooing are controlled, gentle and safe. Strict sterilization and sanitation standards are followed in accordance with OSHA requirements. However, as with any procedure, it's important to make an informed decision that's best for you. Do your research: make absolutely sure your paramedical tattoo artist is reputable, state-licensed and working from a facility which is regulated by the health department.

Tattooing is a non-invasive procedure and generally devoid of any significant adverse effects. However, it does cause microtrauma to the dermis. It may take longer for tattoos to heal in post-radiation treated skin, and for those with autoimmune disorders or for those taking immunosuppressive medication. Diabetics may also take longer to heal. If you are highly sensitive or prone to allergic reactions, a small test spot can be tattooed and monitored to evaluate your body's response. You can also request to see MSDS (material data safety sheets) for the inks used by your paramedical tattoo artist. In rare occasions, people with tattoos and/or permanent makeup have experienced temporary swelling or burning on their tattoos when they underwent magnetic resonance imaging (MRI). If you are scheduled for a MRI, let your physician and MRI tech know about your tattoos (including permanent makeup) so they can ensure a safe imaging procedure.

How many applications are needed?

Many women are fully satisfied with just one session, however, a second session allows me to add some finishing details which can enhance the realism of your nipple-areola portrait. The second session is scheduled 8-10 weeks after your initial session.

How long do paramedical tattoos last?

Tattoos are permanent in that you will always have a permanent marking on your skin. However, a gradual softening of color will occur each year. Many women feel this is advantageous, as they like having the color soften and lighten with time. However, if stronger color is preferred, color enhancement services are always an option. Factors which cause paramedical tattoos to fade are: individual body chemistry, cellular turnover-rejuvenation and exposure to sunlight.

Will insurance cover my post-mastectomy nipple areola tattoos?

The Women's Health and Cancer Rights Act of 1998 requires insurance to cover post-mastectomy reconstruction, including areola/nipple tattooing! Insurance will often reimburse your costs, so please contact your insurance company to discuss this before scheduling your appointment. If the tattoo service is performed at a participating medical center and billed through their office, the paramedical tattoo service should be covered directly by insurance. If the tattoo service is performed at an independent studio location, outside of a medical center, and itemized invoice will be provided to you to submit to your insurance company for reimbursement.

Fortunately, paramedical tattooing is becoming recognized as an integral part of the medical aesthetics genre. Post-mastectomy nipple areola tattoos give back some of what cancer took away and help lift the spirit. This holistic healing is more than skin deep.

Affirmations

"After my diagnosis of breast cancer, a double mastectomy left me struggling to adjust to my new normal. I wanted more than anything to move past those painful moments and find acceptance with my new body... With my new tattoos I caught myself smiling in the mirror. Smiling!!! I no longer saw a body that looked foreign and scarred, instead I saw something beautiful reflecting back..."

— SAMANTHA

"Having had a double mastectomy with reconstruction last year, I did not want a third surgery in nipple reconstruction... My husband watched the entire tattoo procedure and is now fascinated by the art of tattooing. I feel whole again for the first time since my surgery and they look so realistic...I'm a fan of 3D tattoos forever more..."

— MINERVA

" I just love my new tattooed ta-tas! I am so happy to look at my chest and see a beautiful work of art, instead of ugly scars... "

— EVIE

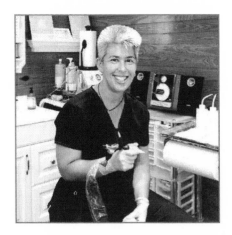

Suzanne Moe was born in Washington, DC to a family serving in the Foreign Service. She was exposed to different cultures and world views from a young age. Suzanne lived in India, Africa and Europe and returned to the United States to earn her degree in Fine Arts from the University of Mary Washington in Fredericksburg, Virginia. After graduating with honors, Suzanne opened a design company which later expanded to include the art form of tattooing. A licensed professional tattoo artist since 1997, Suzanne's current focus is to offer clients the healing, transformational and empowering services of paramedical tattooing with kindness and care. She specializes in 3d nipple/areola tattoos for breast cancer survivors who have undergone mastectomy and are looking for a realistic or artistic completion to their reconstruction.

Suzanne moved to Florida in 2012 and works by appointment from her studio and medical facilities in South Florida.

www.sumaink.com

10

LYMPHEDEMA AND NEUROPATHY

ALEJANDRO BADIA, M.D.

Hand and Upper Limb Problems Related to Breast Cancer

The human hand is a beautifully complex organ of function. It is vital for work, play, and daily life. The shoulder and elbow are critical for placing the hand in space, vital to both earning a living or embracing a loved one.

While several disorders of the hand are primary to that, many dysfunctions can be due to an unrelated problem, such as cancer of the breast and its subsequent treatment. This chapter will be devoted to understanding some of the commonly related problems of the hand and upper extremity as related to breast cancer, as well as delving certain myths and troubling misconceptions. One Australian study showed that over 80% of women suffered from a hand and upper limb disorder following breast cancer treatment.

It is important to see the hand as a confluence of many organ and mechanical systems that come together to provide vital function to its owner. The skeletal system is needed for support and structure with the carpus (wrist), by the far the most complex articulation of the body, comprised of 15 bones and ligaments, powered by muscle tendon units from the forearm and within the hand itself (intrinsic muscles). The vascular system of arteries and veins brings nutrients to the extremity and essentially "keeps it alive". The peripheral nerve system provides that critical touch sensation we all cherish as well as control of fine motor function. The lymphatic system drains the soft tissues of excess fluid and toxins, critical as the most common breast cancer treatment complication attests to. All are wrapped up in the integumentary system (skin) that is outwardly visible to those around us. All systems can be involved as will be discussed.

A review of common upper limb disorders would be incomplete without dispelling some common myths as well. Perhaps because the hand is so vital to the soul, a plethora of misconceptions abound, and it is important to dispel them. Battling breast cancer and the treatment journey is tough enough; no need to saddle the patient with further challenges.

The dreaded complication of lymphedema is notoriously misunderstood, naturally to the afflicted patient, but even to the medical community itself. While 1/3 to ½ of all patients undergoing lymph node dissection as part of breast cancer work-up or treatment may develop this problem, it is impossible to predict who and even when. Some cases can develop decades after surgery, often instigated by minimal trauma, although most times it develops in a delayed manner, usually from 1 to 5 years after the procedure.

The lymphatic system, as previously mentioned, is tasked with transporting the protein-rich interstitial fluid back to the circulatory system through a series of lymph vessels and nodes. The latter filter this fluid, trapping bacteria, cancer cells and viruses, hence the term "swollen glands" which generally portends that the body is fighting some unwanted invader. Lymphedema occurs when that lymph fluid accumulates naturally, leading to swollen soft tissues often accompanied by pain, numbness and a feeling of tightness. This can occur in the hand, entire upper limb, or even the breast and abdomen, depending on the surgery performed and ancillary treatments. This fluid builds up in the spaces between the skin, fat, muscle, vessels and nerves hence leading to the clinical problems so often encountered.

The clinical signs of lymphedema include:

- A heavy and numb feeling in the arm
- Diffuse swelling and achiness
- Tightness of the skin
- Clothing, rings, watch and jewelry feel tight
- Decreased motion of joints in the hand, elbow and shoulder
- Redness, warmth, fever and exquisite tenderness, which can be signs of infection

The definitive diagnosis of lymphedema is difficult but generally three physical measures are used:

1. Circumferential measures at various anatomic landmarks along the limb
2. Volumetric measurements where the limb is submerged in liquid
3. Soft-tissue tonometry where the tissue compression can be quantified.

There are diagnostic studies as well involving CT, MRI, Opto-electric scanning and Lymphoscintigraphy which can all provide some quantitative assessment of the anatomy to help establish the diagnosis. Ultimately, the diagnosis tends to be clinical and perhaps the most common definition of a 2-centimeter difference of arm girth is as useful as any other method for assessment.

The challenge with clinicians has been to recognize who is at risk and of course, how to prevent or minimize it. Risk factors are obviously extensive lymph node removal, but also radiation therapy, adjunctive steroid treatment, and obesity.

However, early treatments that can avoid or at least mitigate the chance of developing this condition are available. Some of these recommendations are perhaps more "urban legend" and will be discussed shortly in a more scientific context.

- Take measures to minimize post-surgical swelling including strict hand elevation, perform prescribed exercises and incorporate use of the arm in ADLs (activities of daily living) as soon as possible.
- Avoid infections and burns by moisturizing skin, minimizing needle sticks in that extremity, and keeping the hand clean. Use antibacterial creams in any at risk areas such as a hangnail, insect bites or mild scrapes.
- Protect the limb from even minor trauma with measures such as wearing a sewing thimble, donning oven mitts in kitchen and protective gloves for chores/gardening and using an electric shaver, not a razor.
- Cold is preferable to hot. Bathing or doing dishes with hot water, using a heating pad, and doing deep tissue massage all signal the body to deliver additional fluid to the compromised area, worsening the condition or perhaps triggering it.
- Avoid pressure or squeezing of the extremity by wearing loose clothes, avoiding carrying heavy shoulder bags or objects, and taking blood pressure readings from opposite arm. This is in sharp contrast with specially fitted compressive sleeves designed to push lymph back to the core. Your physicians may refer you to a specific lymphedema specialist for this and other treatment modalities.
- Commonsense measures of abstaining from smoking, avoiding alcohol, controlling blood sugar, and keeping body weight in check are all vital.

Clearly, taking measures to avoid lymphedema or to minimize its aggravation are critical but once it is established, the affected patient will need well defined guidelines on actual treatment. It is important to understand that a "complete cure" is unlikely due to the under-lying anatomic pathology but getting the condition to a manageable point is a worthwhile goal within reach.

- Exercises that encourage lymph drainage were mentioned as we discussed methods to prevent development. Once established, however, any light exercises that cause contraction of muscles in the limb are helpful and can be taught by a certified lymphedema specialist. Wrapping compressive bandages will also be a mainstay of treatment. This will be taught by the lymphedema specialist as well and may include use of a pneumatic compression device that will intermittently inflate a specially fitted sleeve via a pump, such as Flexitouch® and others, allowing passive treatment that can be done at home alone.
- Special massage techniques known as "manual lymph drainage" are often used and should be done by a lymphedema therapist that is specially trained in this technique. These therapists can often help you obtain a custom compression garment and instruct you in donning and doffing the device so that it is most effective.
- A combined approach of manual therapy with specific compression garments is known as "Complex Decongestive Therapy" (CDT) and is an intense program for more resistant cases where the patient will need to qualify as a candidate. This is administered by therapists with even more rigorous certification as can be obtained by the Norton School of Lymphatic Therapy and other organizations.
- Medical treatments such as diuretics are not effective in high-protein types of edemas such as lymphedema. They

can temporarily mobilize the water, but rapid re-accumulation occurs due to the increased proteins in the interstitial (between cells) space. Benzopyrones are a class of drugs that stimulate macrophage activity, literally removing excess proteins that can decrease edema fluid. However, these effects are modest, inconsistent at best, and significant side effects have been reported such as liver toxicity and even death.

- Surgical treatments are mentioned for completeness sake, but none of them have been clinically successful as a whole. They are divided in two main categories: Physiologic and Reductive. The former is an approach that tries to restore lymphatic flow, either by bringing in tissue with normal lymph mechanics, or by directing microsurgical reattachment of lymph channels to the venous system. Neither has been successful except in anecdotal cases. Reductive procedures are aimed at simply reducing limb girth to a more functional size. This often involves removing tissue and reconstructing with skin grafts or flaps or even using liposuction. While they may reduce limb size, none has been able to correct the underlying physiologic problem.

Given limitations in definitive treatment, and being unable to completely prevent the condition, it is perhaps most important to dispel myths and focus on what seems to work, avoiding a nihilistic approach.

Avoidance of needle sticks seems to be the most misunderstood of common recommendations. This concept originates from the erroneous principle that infection was the underlying cause for swelling of the arm after breast cancer surgery – as espoused by the famous general surgeon, Halstead, in the early 1920s. In fact, there is only one study that supports a potential link between needle sticks and infection and apparently has become the genesis for the broad recommendation regarding venipuncture and breast cancer patients post axillary node dissection. A multitude of studies have shown that intravenous procedures have posed very little risk of any complications, including lymphedema, in the arm having undergone prior surgery including lymph node excision.

The general recommendation of avoiding pressure on the affected limb, such as blood pressure monitoring or tight clothing, also has little scientific support. Furthermore, several studies involving hand surgeons showed no increased complications by using a pneumatic tourniquet on the limb for elective upper limp surgery. A level 4 study demonstrated no new cases of lymphedema or long-term worsening of symptoms in elective hand surgery after a history of axillary lymph node dissection for breast cancer. Anecdotally, I personally cannot recall a single episode of aggravation of the condition having done a variety of upper limb surgeries in these patients, even including fractures of the distal radius that required plate fixation. Carpal tunnel releases are very common, due the ubiquitous nature of the problem, and have had equally successful results in this patient population. In fact, the condition may be more common in these patients for a variety of reasons and deserves the same successful treatment intervention. Since tourniquet use is generally involved, this supports the concept that external compression is not significant risk factor in development of lymphedema. Furthermore, since hand surgery involves making incisions with subsequent wound healing needs, the violation of skin and soft tissue integrity also appears to not be associated with risk of lymphedema or its long-term aggravation.

The practice of elevating the limb long term and avoiding air travel are also lacking objective evidence. Wearing a compressive device during prolonged air travel makes good sense but the actual act of flying likely causes little adversity.

The effect of heat on lymphedema has generally been considered detrimental, but there are even some studies paradoxically showing a positive effect. The same goes for superficial sunburns as patients often avoid sun exposure to an exaggerated degree due to this unfounded concern.

The avoidance of exercise has also been touted since increased blood flow could theoretically lead to increased lymphatic fluid production. Multiple studies have now, fortunately, disproved this concept and even shown that the exercise group, compared to control, demonstrate a decreased incidence of exacerbations of lymphedema and decreased symptoms as well.

It is clear, however, that obesity IS a significant risk factor for development of lymphedema in the post-axillary node dissection patient. The cellular mechanism for this is largely unknown but appears to be related to the fact that a heavier limb will act as a reservoir for lymphatic fluid. With clear understanding and a motivated patient, the avoidance and treatment of obesity appears to be a very manageable risk factor in the development of this difficult complication.

Shoulder and arm stiffness is a relatively common side-effect of ipsilateral (same-side) breast cancer treatment. The cause can be multi-factorial and early intervention with physical/occupational therapy is critical. While scar contracture, adhesions and pain are obvious cause of post-treatment stiffness, a less understood cause is idiopathic adhesive capsulitis of the shoulder. This is a poorly understood condition that is already seen much more commonly in woman, perhaps related to hormonal/metabolic causes, but can be brought on by interventions near the shoulder girdle such as axillary node dissection, radical mastectomy or even simple lumpectomy. Avoidance by early physiotherapy is key but established "frozen shoulder" needs a more focused approach often including articular injection of corticosteroid and even arthroscopic capsular release. The latter can often be avoided by aggressive approach, however this simple, outpatient, minimally invasive approach should not be delayed in the patient progressing poorly as it generally leads to nearly complete resolution.

Nerve disorders related to breast cancer treatment are also relatively common and can be some of the most severe symptoms, as well as challenging to clearly diagnose. Early evaluation by a hand and peripheral nerve surgeon is critical, often in conjunction with an electrophysiologist specializing in nerve conduction evaluations.

Nerve symptoms may appear immediately after surgery or in months following certain treatments such as axillary radiation. The key is early recognition and intervention although some disorders unfortunately have little remedy and patient counseling is paramount.

Chemotherapy-induced peripheral neuropathy is a troubling complication of many cancers due to the neurotoxic effects of many treatment regimens. This typically occurs with drugs within the taxane, vinca alkaloid and platinum groups. The platinum analogue Cisplatin has a notoriously high neurotoxic effect and risk of neuropathy is higher in patients with previous treatment or underlying neuropathies or radiculopathy (nerve root compression). Most of these neuropathies are sensory, therefore the symptoms are troubling (numbness, tingling) but muscle weakness is rarely associated. Treatment involves education, therapy and certain medications that mediate the effects of the agent including anticonvulsants and antidepressants.

As mentioned, cervical radiculopathy (pinched nerve in neck) can worsen in setting of chemotherapy regimens or patients after breast surgery and/or radiation treatment. Physiotherapy, NSAIDs (non-steroidal anti-inflammatories) and oral/injected steroids can all have major beneficial effect. Persistent symptoms are very amenable to surgical treatment if a focal nerve root compression can be diagnosed clearly, usually due to degenerative changes, ruptured disc or occasionally tumor growth in extreme cases.

Pain in the upper arm or axilla can be due to a post-mastectomy pain syndrome, usually from scarring or damage of nerves in the area of breast/axilla surgery, most commonly the intercostobrachial nerve. This should be differentiated from Phantom Breast Syndrome (PBS) where patients can have pain perceived in the breast area, or arm, even though the breast has been removed. Treatment strategies include physiotherapy modalities focused on skin desensitization and promoting nerve healing.

Brachial plexopathy can lead to diffuse dysfunction in both upper limb sensory and motor function. The brachial plexus is a confluence of nerves that are compromised of cervical nerve roots that come together to then create a multitude of nerves, including the 3 major nerves to the upper limb, radial, ulnar and median. The plexus can be scarred or injured by radiation therapy, tumor growth infiltration or even neurotoxicity from chemo agents as previously mentioned.

The probability of radiation induced brachial plexopathy is related to the dose per fraction and then total dose received and is beyond the scope of this chapter. Vast improvements in this treatment modality have led to a decreased incidence, but the most severe cases will need medication for pain "control" as well as specific physiotherapy. Surgery for brachial plexus is disorders is challenging as is in the obstetric and post-traumatic etiologies, therefore radiation induced plexopathies that progress are often untreatable. Fortunately, many of these spontaneously resolve and patients will be closely followed.

The last category of nerve related disorders is known as compression neuropathies. One of them, carpal tunnel syndrome, is perhaps the best known but most commonly misunderstood malady affecting the hand and upper limb. Some studies have shown that nearly 10% of women can suffer from this common median nerve compression disorder, and because breast cancer is generally a female affliction, some relationships have been surmised. There is little doubt that many upper limb disorders can initiate or cause carpal tunnel syndrome to progress and become symptomatic to the point that surgical treatment is necessary. Fortunately, median nerve decompression at the wrist is perhaps the most successful and reproducible procedure that any hand surgeon performs on routine basis.

The median nerve, along with 9 flexor tendons, sits within a tunnel 2 centimeters long that is bound by small carpal (wrist) bones and the roof is a thick ligament called the transverse carpal ligament, or flexor retinaculum. Compression of the nerve usually occurs due to thickening of the accompanying flexor tendons or their surrounding sheaths (flexor tenosynovium). Therefore, any metabolic or hormonal alteration that can affect the sheath matrix may lead to a secondary nerve compression. This can be seen in conditions such as diabetes, gout, hypothyroidism or even the 3rd trimester of pregnancy. Alterations of estrogen balances are obviously part of menopause; hence many women will begin to suffer from CTS symptoms in their 4th and 5th decades. Therefore, CTS may simply be an underlying issue and not at all related to the development of breast cancer or even its myriad of treatments.

Cubital tunnel syndrome, compression of the ulnar nerve at the elbow, is also a relatively common condition of the upper limb. This is where the ulnar nerve ("funny bone") at the elbow is compressed or irritated. Therefore, it stands to reason that any alteration to the upper limb including lymphedema, peripheral neuropathy, or proximal scarring can trigger the symptoms of CTS or hasten the progression of this and other compression neuropathies. Early evaluation by a hand surgeon is important and can be the least troubling complication related to cancer of the breast and its treatment.

Breast cancer is obviously a very devastating diagnosis to a woman, her family and surrounding social network. Treatment advances have made this a now often curable condition. Secondary problems of the hand and upper extremity, as discussed in this treatise, require early detection and intervention, often within the realm of the upper limb specialist. Frequently, patients do not know where to seek specific help within the musculoskeletal realm and therefore orthopedic walk-in centers (OrthoNOW®, DOC etc.) have begun to emerge within the medical care infrastructure. Careful discussion with the lead physicians (PCP and breast oncologist) can sort out many of these complaints and the orthopedic subspecialist will play a supporting role. Breast cancer patients will face many challenges but maintaining a functioning and relatively pain free upper limb will surely contribute to optimal quality of life.

~

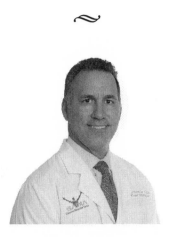

Alejandro Badia, MD, FACS is a hand and upper extremity surgeon at Badia Hand to Shoulder Center in Doral, Florida previously serving as chief of hand surgery, Baptist Hospital of Miami. Dr. Badia studied physiology at Cornell University and obtained his medical degree at NYU, where he also trained in orthopedics. A hand fellowship at Alleghany General Hospital in Pittsburgh was followed by an AO trauma fellowship in Freiburg, Germany. He runs an active international hand fellowship, serves on the editorial board of two hand journals, and previously organized a yearly Miami meeting for surgeons /therapists devoted to upper limb arthroscopy and arthroplasty. This international meeting was held at the world-renowned Miami Anatomical Research Center (M.A.R.C.), the world's 2nd largest surgical cadaveric training lab which Dr. Badia co-founded in 2005. He is a founding member of the American Hand Institute, a think tank and medical device start-up company focused on minimally invasive solutions to hand, wrist and elbow pathology.

In 2008, Dr. Badia completed the Badia Hand to Shoulder Center, a fully integrated clinical facility for the upper limb also encompassing the Surgery Center at Doral, a rehabilitation center, and an MRI imaging facility. In 2010, Dr. Badia inaugurated OrthoNOW®, the first immediate orthopedic care center in South Florida. It is staffed by surgeons from the International Orthopedic Group (IOG), a group of surgeons from lower extremity, upper limb and spine subspecialties who also treat elective orthopedic problems in international patients. OrthoNOW® was officially franchised in early 2013 and is actively engaging healthcare entrepreneurs and surgeons, here and abroad to open orthopedic urgent care facilities in the United States and around the world.

Dr. Badia is past worldwide president of the International Society for Sport Traumatology of the Hand (ISSPORTH), was named to 100 Latinos Miami, has been given legacy awards by several organizations and was featured on the Hispanic Entrepreneur website. He is a member of multiple national subspecialty medical societies (AAOS, ASSH, AAHS), and honorary member of more than 10 international hand surgery and arthroscopy associations. He served as honored professor at the prestigious Philadelphia Hand Course in 2012. Dr. Badia has lectured on all six continents and is currently focused on improving healthcare delivery in the orthopedics and sports medicine realm.

He can be easily reached via www.drbadia.com, a patient education portal and website for hand surgeon academic exchange, or via (305) 227-HAND at the Badia Hand to Shoulder Center or at OrthoNOW®, (305) 537-7272, www.OrthoNOWcare.com.

11

CARDIAC EFFECTS AFTER BREAST CANCER TREATMENT

JAVIER JIMENEZ, M.D.

Determining the cardiovascular risk in cancer survivor

Cancer therapies such as chemotherapy and radiation therapy are associated to potential risks of developing cardiovascular complications. As a matter of fact, cardiac complications are one of the most common side effects of these medications. It is important to understand the stage at which medical interventions are applied when it refers to cardiac disease. It is important to identify patients that prior to cancer therapy are already at higher risk to develop cardiac complications such as pre-existing diabetes or hypertension. In those, mitigating the effect of those underlying conditions by optimizing their medical therapy is essential. During cancer therapy, monitoring to identify known cardiovascular complications mainly associated to chemotherapy are required to avoid dose interruptions or discontinuation. After cancer therapy and for an indefinite period, survivors will also require a different type of surveillance for late cardiovascular effects to improve long term health. (1)

In 2012, there were 13.7 million adult cancer survivors in the United States. Cancer survival continues to improve and most children with cancer will become adults. (2). In a study by Patkail et al, of those women who died because of cardiovascular disease, 25.5% were categorized as having cardiovascular disease as a comorbid condition at the time of their breast cancer diagnosis. Conversely, of those women who had cardiovascular disease as a comorbid condition at the time of their breast cancer diagnosis and who died during the study period, 41.9% died from cardiovascular disease. (3). Under-diagnoses and under-treatment of cardiac conditions may be important issues for women diagnosed with cancer, as their cancer diagnosis can be perceived by both the patient and her caregivers as the overriding medical priority.

In general, cardiac complications are best categorized are those related to chemotherapy and those related to radiation therapy. In both categories, one can describe early and late presentations. Sometimes, cardiac complications occur or become enhanced from having had both chemotherapy and radiation therapies combined.

Chemotherapy induced cardiotoxicity

There are different types of toxicity induced by cancer treatment with chemotherapy.

Heart failure, a condition that leads to fluid congestion and inability of the heart to pump properly, is associated to chemotherapy drugs such as anthracyclines, Cytoxan, HER2/neu-inhibitors and VEGF-inhibitors. This can result in a decompensated cardiomyopathy. Another common cardiac complication are arrhythmias, which are irregular or fast heart rhythms, commonly associated to taxanes such as paclitaxel, and docetaxel. Vascular disease such as hypertension and vasculitis, an inflammation of the blood vessels, occur with 5FU and platinum-based agents (4).

The most obvious chemotherapy-related cardiac effect on the heart is weakening of the heart. Cardiotoxicity has been defined based on the presence of heart failure signs and symptoms of heart failure. The ejection fraction, a parameter to quantitate the contractility of the heart muscle is often used in cardiac imaging. Certain definitions of cardiotoxicity include a decrease in the heart contractility or a decrease of the ejection fraction by 5% below 55% with heart failure symptoms or by 10% below 50% without symptoms. The American society of Echocardiography and the European Association of Imaging define cardiotoxicity by a drop of the ejection fraction greater that 10% below 53%. There are two types of cardiotoxicity: type I, associated to anthracyclines, where there is permanent death of the myocytes or heart muscle cells and type II; associated to trastuzumab, where the myocyte damage is reversible. (5,6)

Doxorubicin is one of the most common used anthracyclines. It is associated to the development of heart dysfunction in 5% of those patients that receive a cumulative dose greater than 4 mg/m2 but increases to 48% when the dose is greater than 700 mg/m2. Anthracycline toxicity shows a dose dependent effect. The risk of heart failure increases substantially with cumulative doses greater than 250 mg/m2. There are also different onsets of toxicity related to anthracyclines; acute -within 2 weeks; early on -within one year and late - years or decades after treatment. Since most cases occur within the first year after treatment, early detection becomes crucial for preservation of the ejection fraction. Acute toxicity most likely presents with development of cardiac arrhythmias, electrocardiographic changes, morphological heart dysfunction and symptoms of heart failure (8,9)

Risk factors associated to the development of anthracycline cardiotoxicity are: cumulative dose, female gender, older patients, renal insufficiency, previous radiation, other chemotherapy given in association and preexisting cardiac conditions.

Transtuzuman, a chemotherapy agent commonly used as adjuvant therapy, produces a cardiotoxicity which is not dose dependent and is reversible for the most part. It is more commonly seen in those patients that were previously treated with anthracycline, have history of hypertension, are older and obese. The incidence of transtuzumab cardiac toxicity can be reduced by staging the administration of transtuzumab after anthracycline or by providing anthracycline free regimens. These strategies should be considered early in the treatment to avoid unnecessary interruptions or discontinuation of chemotherapy (7).

Drugs that inhibit the vascular endothelial growth factor signaling pathway (VEGF) can produce both reversible and irreversible cardiac complications between 3-15% of the patients, although the impact and prognosis difficult to ascertain since these drugs are introduced in more advanced cancer stages.

Other chemotherapeutic agents can produce heart dysfunction such as cisplatin, ifosfamide, cyclophosphamide and taxanes.

Chemotherapy agents can develop other forms of cardiovascular disease such as coronary ischemia, cardiac arrhythmias, blood clots and development of severe arterial hypertension.

Detection of cardiotoxicity

Cardiotoxicity may present with or without signs and symptoms, however it is not advisable to wait until symptoms develop to diagnose cardiotoxicity. The use of early cardiac imaging has proved an ideal strategy to detect subtle morphological changes that would indicate development of an early cardiomyopathy (10). Three cardiac imaging techniques are currently available. Echocardiography, Multigated Acquisition Scan (MUGA) and cardiac magnetic resonance imaging (MRI). Each type of imaging has its benefits and disadvantages (See Table 1). In addition to cardiac imaging, biomarkers, which are laboratory tests that measure elevation of cardiac products in blood, such as troponins and brain natriuretic peptides also serve to indicate early cardiac damage. A combination of cardiac imaging and biomarkers have proved to be superior than each strategy alone. Evaluation of risk should include a careful physical examination, understanding existing co morbidities and baseline data that would include assessment of cardiac function with cardiac imaging and obtaining baseline biomarkers (11,12,13,18).

Table 1

	Advantages	Disadvantages	Modalities
Echocardiogram	Easily available	Variable interpretation	3D
	Measure of pressures	Variable image window	2D
	No radiation	Variable equipment	Strain imaging
Nuclear imaging	Minimal variability	Radiation	SPECT
			MUGA
Magnetic Resonance	Accurate	Procedure length	MRI/MRA
		Enclosure	T1/T2 images

The frequency of evaluation of cardiac function may vary with the type of chemotherapy agent that was used. For anthracyclines, a baseline and end-of-therapy assessment should be performed. In those where high doses of anthracyclines are used, earlier imaging is recommended when reaching doses of 240 mg/m2 or higher. In patients treated with anti-HER2 chemotherapy, a baseline evaluation of cardiac function, every 3 months and after treatment should be followed. Patients treated with VEGF inhibitors should be evaluated earlier, typically 2-4 weeks, specially in those with higher risk or every 4 cycles for those at lower risk.

Detection of coronary artery disease

The development of coronary insufficiency or coronary artery disease occurs because of vasospasm and vessel thrombosis with or without associated underlying or premature atherosclerosis. Several drugs have been reported to be associated to ischemic complications such us 5-FU, cisplatin, VEGF inhibitors but also after radiation therapy. Usually patients develop symptoms of chest pain or angina. In women angina like symptoms may be atypical, and a higher index of suspicion is warranted. Exercise or pharmacological stress tests, in combination with cardiac imaging (Stress echo, nuclear stress test) are usually the first line testing, however cardiac catheterization or coronary CT angiography may be required to better define the coronary anatomy. There are different ways to restore normal coronary flow in area compromised by a blood clot or a blockage such as coronary artery bypass or catheter-based procedures.

Detection of valvular disease

Valvular disease, described more commonly as valvular lesions that lead to narrowing or leaking of the cardiac valves, is not usually related to chemotherapy rather by radiation therapy.

Detection of arrhythmias

Cardiac arrhythmias may present as slow or fast heart rhythms. They usually occur in the context of direct myocardial cell toxicity or direct effect of myocardial cell electrophysiology. Drugs associated are like those that cause myocardial toxicity and other drug classes such as histone deacetylase inhibitors and tyrosine kinase inhibitors. Cardiac arrhythmias can be detected by the placement of short term (Holter monitor) or long-term (telemetry or post event monitors). Arrhythmias can be categorized as benign or malignant. Common relatively benign arrhythmias are atrial fibrillation, premature ventricular beats, sinus tachycardia which are usually treated with medications. Lethal arrhythmias such as ventricular tachycardia or ventricular fibrillation may occur when the heart function diminishes or when electrical changes occur in the electrocardiogram that predisposes the heart to these arrhythmias. Prevention, by sequential electrocardiogram (ECG) monitoring is recommended in those patients at risk.

Detection of arterial hypertension

Arterial hypertension is a common condition, however certain drugs, more commonly VEGF inhibitors are known to develop arterial hypertension de novo or to exacerbate underlying hypertension. when it develops, it should be treated following practice guidelines.

Untreated high blood pressure may result in an additive risk to develop cardiotoxicity. Drugs such as angiotensin converting enzyme inhibitors (ACEI), angiotensin receptor blockers (ARB), beta blockers and calcium channel blockers are commonly used to treat hypertension.

Detection of thromboembolism

Venous and arterial blood clot embolism is increased in patient with underlying cancer. Venous embolism is much more common, up to 20% of cancer patients that require hospitalization. Older patients with multiple comorbidities and undergoing major surgeries are at the highest risk. No specific chemotherapy drugs except VEGF inhibitors are known to increase the risk of thrombotic embolism. Prophylactic anticoagulation with unfractionated heparin or low molecular weight heparin are recommended to most hospitalized cancer patients to avoid venous thromboembolism.

Radiation therapy

Radiation therapy is used as adjuvant therapy in most cancer patients and in many patients treated with breast cancer. Cardiac complications related to thoracic radiation have been well described. Although current radiation doses are generally lower and better localized than before; doses greater than 30 Gy may cause direct heart damage. This injury may affect different heart structures such as the pericardium; the membrane surrounding the heart, coronary arteries, conduction system, valves and myocardial cells. Pericardial fibrosis is a late complication (>10 years) that may occur in 10% of the patients receiving thoracic radiation. It involves thickening and scarring of the pericardium. This condition may present with symptoms like heart failure; congestion and edema. The treatment is difficult and may require surgical stripping of the pericardium. Coronary artery disease or narrowing of the arteries that supply the heart can affect small and large vessels of the heart circulation. It is more common in patients that have received thoracic radiation at high doses. Periodic screening is recommended, specially in those patients with underlying cardiac risk factors who underwent radiation that involved the heart. There is no consensus when to start screening for coronary artery disease in patients that have received thoracic radiation; however, in patient over 45 years old, screening have been suggested to start 5 years after radiation at 5 year intervals. This screening if perform through regular stress testing. Valvular disease leading to narrowing and insufficiency if the heart valves and direct myocardial injury (restrictive cardiomyopathy more commonly) related to radiation can occur as a late complication of radiation therapy. Valvular disease is easily identified using echocardiography. Risk factors to development radiation related cardiac complication are younger age at the time of radiation administration, higher dose of radiation, heart exposure to radiation, longer interval since radiation and adjuvant chemotherapy (15).

Prevention of cardiac damage

As a rule, identifying and optimizing treatment of known cardiovascular risk factors such as hypertension, diabetes and hyperlipidemia are first line interventions to prevent cardiac complications. In addition, exercise and diet contribute to the general well-being prior or during cancer treatment. There are several drugs used in cardiovascular disease, that applied in the setting of suspected chemotherapy induced cardiotoxicity may prevent late onset cardiotoxicity. For example, in patients that develop abnormal troponins after high dose chemotherapy, if treated with an ACEI inhibitor (captopril) prevented from a decrease of heart function and dilatation of the heart (16). In patients at high risk of chemotherapy induced cardiomyopathy, early treatment with enalapril seems to prevent cardiotoxicity (14). In other studies, the addition of a beta blocker (metoprolol or bisoprolol) to ACEI attenuated the potential decline of chemotherapy induced cardiomyopathy. The earlier after identifying myocardial damage the better outcome when using these medications. Dexarazoxane, an iron chelating agent, can prevent myocardial dysfunction when administered in conjunction with doxorubicin. There are several position papers that establish recommendations of medical therapy in certain situations with the purpose to minimize cardiac damage. There are numerous medical and non-medical publications that recommend specific diets and types of exercise to improve outcomes in cancer patients. In general, is difficult to recommend any of them, however, everyone can understand the concept of a healthy diet and that exercise entails a physical effort. For healthy and sick individuals diet and exercise improves longevity and quality of life while increasing the chances of a healthier lifetime.

Cardio-oncology, a new specialty within cardiology

In recent years, a cardio-oncology has started to shape as an incipient sub-specialty amongst cardiologists. Cardio-oncology aims to improve and standardize medical care for patient treated for cancer who are at risk for cardiac disease or develop cardiovascular complication. Cardio-oncology services are developing across the United States as demand for specialized treatment of cardiac complications related to cancer treatment is increasing. This close collaboration between cardiology and oncology physicians in specialized centers will help applying best clinical practices to achieve improved long-term survival of cancer patients. Cardio-oncology currently is not a designated a designated American Board of Internal Medicine cardiology sub-specialty. Different cardiologist tends gravitate to incorporate cardio-oncology in their practice such as those already boarded in Echocardiography, Nuclear Cardiology or Advanced Heart Failure Transplant. Clinical experience and commitment to this area is what matters most when it relates to choosing a cardiac specialist to the cancer team.

In summary, cancer patients require treatments with chemotherapy and radiation that can develop early and late cardiac complications. Prevention, early recognition and prompt management leads to improve outcomes and survival. Oncology teams that incorporate a cardiac specialist familiar with cardio oncology is an advantage for the optimal care of cancer patients.

I acknowledge the participation of Tina Hyman R.N. in the writing and technical editing of this chapter.

References

1. Armernian et al. *Journal of Clinical Oncology* 35, no. 8 (March 10 2017) 893-911.
2. www.cancer.gov/about-cancer/understanding/statistics
3. Patnaik JL et al. Breast Cancer Res. 2011 Jun 20;13(3):R64.
4. Lenneman CG , Sawyer DM, Circ Res. 2016 Mar 18;118(6):1008-20.
5. Bird BR, Swain SM Clin Cancer Res. 2008 Jan 1;14(1):14-24.
6. Yancy C.W. et al. Circulation. 2017;136:e137-e161
7. Ewer MS and Ewer SM. Nat Rev Cardiol. 2015. 12. 547-58
8. Ewer MS. Nat Rev Cardiol. 12; 547-558 2015
9. Armenian SH et al. Blood. 2011 Dec 1;118(23):6023-9.
10. Cardinale D. et al. Circulation. 2015 Jun 2;131(22):1981-8.
11. Khouri MG et al. Circulation. 2012; 126: 2749-63
12. Blessberger H and Binder T. Heart 2010; 96:716-22
13. Plana JC et al. Eur Heart J – CV Imaging 2014. 15(1063-93)
14. *Cardinale et al. Circulation. 2006;114:2474-2481*
15. Groarke J.D. et al. *European Heart Journal*, Volume 35, Issue 10, 7 March 2014, Pages 612–623
16. Zamorano J.L, Lancelloti P. et al. *European Heart Journal*, Volume 37, Issue 36, 21 September 2016, Pages 2768–2801
17. Barac A. et al. JACC Vol 65, I 25, June 2015. 2739-2746.
18. 18. Plana J.C. et al. J Am Soc Echocardiogra 2014: 27 :911-39.

~

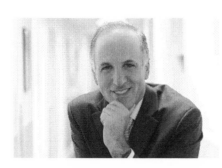

Dr. Javier Jimenez is currently the Director of Advanced Heart Failure and Pulmonary Hypertension at the Miami Cardiac and Vascular Institute, Baptist Health South. He a Clinical Associate Professor of Medicine at the Hebert Wertheim College of Medicine at Florida International University.

He obtained his medical degree and Ph.D. at the University of Alcala de Henares in Madrid, Spain. Dr. Jimenez then fulfilled an Internal Medicine Residency and Cardiology Fellowship at Brown University in Providence, Rhode Island and completed additional fellowships in Advanced Heart Failure/Cardiac Transplantation at the Cleveland Clinic, Ohio and in Interventional Cardiology at Brown University. Dr Jimenez has published extensively and participated in multiple national and international clinical trials.

Dr. Jimenez is Board Certified in Internal Medicine, Cardiology, Interventional Cardiology, Nuclear Cardiology, Echocardiography and Advanced Heart Failure and Cardiac Transplantation. He is a Fellow member of the American College of Cardiology and American Society of Nuclear Cardiology. He is currently a member of the American Society of Echocardiography and the Heart Failure Society of America.

You can reach him at (305) 666-4633 or jjimenez@smiamiheart.com.

12

PAIN MANAGEMENT

DENNIS PATIN, M.D.

It is hard to believe that more than seven years have passed since the initial publication of *The Empty Cup Runneth Over*. It is an honor for me to have been asked to write a follow up chapter on anesthesia and pain management. The name of the original chapter was *Reaching Nirvana – Pain, Pain, Go Away – Anesthesia Saves the Day*. While that title remains appropriate, in this updated chapter I will seek to incorporate additional information on advances made in the field and how those advances have led to a safer and more pleasant experience for a woman undergoing any type of diagnostic or surgical procedure related to a potential or actual cancer diagnosis. Also, we will discuss contemporary pain management in the acute and chronic setting.

Anesthesia literally means "without sensation," and is generally referred to as a service or treatment a patient may receive to allow a diagnostic or surgical procedure to take place without discomfort. Discomfort can be emotional or physical. Emotional discomfort can be alleviated by reducing anxiety, and by providing amnesia for the procedure. This is the building block or base of anesthetic care, and it starts with the anesthesia care provider-patient relationship.

Before any procedure, you will have a meeting with that provider, where you'll have an opportunity to ask questions about your anesthetic and the choices you may have. This anesthesia care provider could be your doctor, administering local anesthetic and/or sedative medications, or it could be a physician anesthesia specialist known as an anesthesiologist, working alone or with the help of an anesthetist known as a CRNA (Certified Registered Nurse Anesthetist) or AA (Anesthesiologist Assistant) a type of PA (Physician Assistant). Such a care team is quite common, and is believed to be associated with superior outcomes, especially in more complicated cases. A good discussion of anesthesia options goes a long way toward building trust and minimizing anxiety.

Very minor procedures may require only local anesthesia, which is typically injected into the site where a needle biopsy on incisional biopsy is to take place. The local anesthesia literally "numbs" the area for hours, wearing off gradually. Depending on physician, institution, and patient preference, the local anesthesia may be supplemented by oral or intravenous sedative medications designed to relieve anxiety and provide amnesia. These can be administered by or under the supervision of the physician performing the procedure, where it is known as Sedation/Analgesia, or by the anesthesia care team specialists, where it is known as MAC or (Monitored Anesthesia Care). MAC is typically used for more invasive or painful procedures, in patients who have more complex medical conditions, and in those where simple local anesthesia is insufficient.

General anesthesia is administered for more complex and painful procedures, and only by the anesthesia care team. In addition to the reduction of anxiety and procedural amnesia, a benefit of general anesthesia is absence of sensation, absence of pain, absence of movement, and reduction in abnormal reflexes during the procedure. The anesthesia care team will monitor and support your vital signs continuously, often with the aid of a breathing tube inserted after you are asleep and taken out just before you return to full consciousness.

A common fear is awareness under anesthesia, that the patient will remember parts of their procedure and be unable to signal or notify their anesthesia care provider. Fortunately, the incidence of this is extremely low. If you are particularly concerned, mention it to your provider and special steps will be taken to further minimize the risk.

Modern-day anesthesia is very safe, so safe that malpractice premiums for anesthesiologists are similar to that of general medical doctors such as internists and family physicians. Contributing to that safety is a preoperative evaluation, where your medical history, surgical history, medications, and allergies are reviewed, indicated laboratory and diagnostic tests such as an EKG are performed, and conditions are optimized. No patient is too sick to receive anesthesia, and no patient is too healthy not to benefit from the proper anesthetic care for their procedure or condition. During this preoperative evaluation, you will receive instructions regarding which medications to take or stop taking, and how long to fast before the procedure. It helps to have a friend or family member with you, as it can be confusing. For outpatient procedures, you will be asked to have a caregiver take you home.

In the recovery room, you may be given additional pain relievers known as opioid analgesics orally or intravenously, and this treatment may be continued in the inpatient setting with what is known as PCA (Patient Controlled Analgesia). For home use, you may receive a prescription for common oral pain relievers such as morphine, oxycodone (Percocet), hydrocodone (Vicodin), hydromorphone (Dilaudid), and others.

Post-operative or post-procedure discomfort is normal, and will rapidly improve in several days. Any significant pain lasting more than a week or two should be brought to the attention of your surgeon. He or she may then wish to refer you to a pain specialist, a medical doctor with unique knowledge and skills to help you further. After a consultation, the pain specialist may recommend a number of options ranging from acupuncture and physical therapy, to additional medications or procedures such as nerve blocks and injections. Fortunately, the number or percentage of patients undergoing procedures and surgery and later developing pain requiring a pain specialist is very small.

Should you be diagnosed with cancer, there may be associated pain from the tumor itself, or from surgery, chemotherapy, or radiation treatments. The most important thing you can do in this regard is to inform your health care team about your symptoms. They will ask questions to assess your pain in more detail. In fact, pain is considered the "fifth vital sign" after blood pressure, heart rate, respiratory rate, and temperature. Assessing pain is done at all healthcare visits, inpatient and outpatient.

After assessment, several decisions can be made, ranging from no action needed because of minimal pain or patient request to urgent consultation with a pain specialist. A pain specialist is a physician with additional training and experience in the medical specialty of pain management. These physicians are usually also anesthesiologists, neurologists, physical medicine and rehabilitation specialists, or psychiatrists. They can be found in solo practice, group practice settings, or university based academic centers.

A pain specialist will take a more in-depth history, perform a focused pain exam, review medical records, and come up with several treatment plans, ranging from the simplest, to the most involved. Keeping a pain diary may be useful, in addition to involving and bringing a friend or family member to the consultation and follow-up appointments.

Treatments are either considered noninvasive or invasive. All things on the outside of the body are noninvasive; this includes physical therapy, acupuncture, exercise, improving sleep, and psychologic and spiritual support.

Invasive includes anything that goes into the body, and the most common treatment here is medication. Three broad categories of medications are:

1. Nonsteroidal anti-inflammatory medications such as ibuprofen and acetaminophen. They are general

purpose pain relievers and several are available over the counter.

2. Opioids such as morphine, oxycodone (Percocet and Oxycontin), hydromorphone (Dilaudid), oxymorphone (Opana), transdermal fentanyl (Duragesic), buprenorphine (Butrans), tramadol (Ultram), tapentadol (Nucynta), and methadone.

3. Adjuvants. The most common are the anticonvulsants and antidepressants, topical medications, and everything else that doesn't fit the above categories.

Your primary care physician or cancer specialist may start you on some of these medications while reserving others for the pain specialist.

In up to 20% of patients, medical management will be insufficient, either failing to satisfactorily relieve pain or secondary to unacceptable side effects such as sedation. In these cases, selected nerve blocks can be performed or the delivery route of medication changed. A very effective route is intrathecal, also known as intraspinal or neuraxial. Here a small catheter is implanted into the fluid surrounding the spinal cord and the catheter is connected to a delivery system, usually an implanted drug reservoir known as a pump. Pain relief can be substantially better than systemic administration, with a marked reduction in side effects as well.

This is a natural time to discuss the concepts of palliative care and hospice. Palliative care is simply attempting to relieve various symptoms of a disease process that has no cure. Hospice is palliative care at the end of life. Palliative care is a medical specialty like pain management, with various physician specialists receiving additional training. Many, if not most, also work in the hospice field. They are excellent pain management specialists as well, with a slightly different focus and perspective.

In summary, a woman facing a potential cancer diagnosis or actual diagnosis will come to interact with the medical specialties of anesthesiology and pain management. We are all committed to allaying your physical and emotional pain and suffering, no matter where you are on the cancer treatment continuum.

~

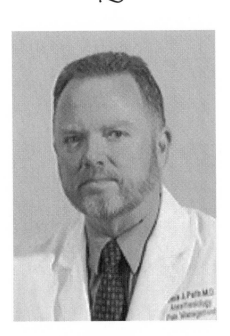

Dennis Patin, M.D. is a specialist in anesthesiology and interventional pain medicine. He earned his M.D. from the University of Miami School of Medicine/Jackson Memorial Hospital in 1985 before completing an internship at Oakland Naval Hospital in 1986, followed by a residency at Jackson Memorial Hospital in 1992. He is an Associate Professor of Clinical Anesthesiology at University of Miami, Miller School of Medicine and is certified by the American Board of Anesthesiology – Pain Medicine. Licensed to treat patients in California and Florida, Dr. Patin currently practices in Miami, Florida and Plantation, Florida.

13

ORAL CARE, CANCER CARE AND YOU: UNDERSTANDING HOW IT ALL COMES TOGETHER

RITA DARGHAM, D.M.D.

Cancer, from the time it is diagnosed to completion of its treatment, is a heart-wrenching experience for all involved. It is a period of tremendous stress and pressure not only for the patients themselves but also for the family and friends supporting the cause. Having participated as a caregiver to various family members who lost their battles to cancer, my father being the dearest to me, I am especially touched by the opportunity to share my thoughts and knowledge with those patients undergoing cancer treatment today. As a practicing restorative, preventive, and cosmetic dentist I am in a unique position to inspire the integration of medicine and dentistry in creating a multidisciplinary approach to the treatment of cancer. My comments in this chapter are based on established studies performed over the recent past, as well as on my own personal and professional experiences with cancer therapies as related to oral health.

Although the American Cancer Society reports that, except for skin cancer, breast cancer is the most common malignancy among American women, most diagnosed with this condition can expect an excellent outcome. That said, a woman undergoing breast cancer treatment today is expected to enjoy a five-year survival rate greater that 80%[1]. With over 200,000 women diagnosed with breast cancer in the United States every year, knowing a majority will benefit from an excellent survival rate, it is imperative to understand how to orchestrate, implement, and maintain short and long-term goals aimed at optimizing quality of life.

Presently, there are more than 2.8 million breast cancer survivors in the United States[1]. Because most women diagnosed with breast cancer can expect an excellent outcome, with a 5-year survival rate above 80%, long term survivorship issues, including those related to oral health, are important components of breast cancer care and follow-up. Helping patients with breast cancer maintain optimal oral health is a key component in the overall continuum of care.

The risk of developing breast cancer increases with age, with approximately 67% of invasive disease diagnosed in women age 55 or older. The average woman has a 12.5% lifetime risk of developing breast cancer. Post-menopausal women make up a majority of diagnosed cases, and approximately 70% of these cancers express the estrogen and/or progesterone receptor and can be treated with anti-estrogen therapy[1].

Risk factors for breast cancer are established. These include:

- Gender
- Family History
- Late Menopause
- Early Menarche
- Ethnicity
- Genetics
- Long Term Hormone Replacement Therapy
- Breast Density

Additionally, studies have shown that increasing alcoholic beverage consumption from one to three drinks per day also increases the risk of breast cancer by 7% to 20%, respectively.

The rationale for breast cancer treatment is complex and based on several prognostic and predictive factors. These may include tumor histology and grade, lymph node involvement, clinical and pathological stage, tumor hormone receptor content, comorbid conditions, menopausal status, age, and patient preference.

Specific breast cancer treatment modalities may include:

- Resective Surgery
- Chemotherapy
- Radiotherapy
- Anti-Estrogen Therapy
- Intravenous Bisphosphonate Administration

Whether selected alone or in combination, acute side effects and long-term complications of breast cancer therapies have a marked impact on the patient's oral health, oral health-related quality of life, and therapy compliance.

Oral health plays a vital role in one's overall quality of life. Unfortunately, cancer therapies such as those mentioned above can deleteriously affect a breast cancer patient's oral health status. Orally related side effects and complications of cancer treatment are often overlooked in clinical practice. It is the responsibility of the entire medical-dental team to fully understand the role cancer therapies play in influencing the oral environment, whether before, during, or after treatment. It is this chapter's aim to draw health care professionals' and patients' attention to oral complications breast cancer patients may experience. Brief comments on contemporary cancer therapies, followed by a description of oral complications associated with these, will be presented. Finally, a summary of preventive strategies and treatment options for common oral complications will be discussed. Coupled with the ongoing advances in cancer detection and treatment modalities, the current and future trend would entail increased likelihood for dentists and the entire oral health team, including the dental hygienist, to encounter patients who are currently, or have previously been, under cancer therapy.

As mentioned previously, contemporary breast cancer treatment modalities include surgical resection, chemotherapy, radiotherapy, anti-estrogen (hormonal) therapy, and the use of IV bisphosphonates, either administered alone or in combination. Although effectiveness of cancer treatment is noted, collateral damage to the head and neck structures is often encountered as an unwanted complication or consequence. Oral complications, be they acute or chronic, may arise throughout and after cancer treatment. Poorly restored dentition, moderate to advanced periodontal disease, and other pathologies associated with negligence or oral health care, may be significantly worsened by the many oral complications resulting from aggressive cancer treatment, greatly hampering patients' quality of life. OPTIMAL ORAL HEALTH IS IMPERATIVE! Maintaining optimal oral health is essential in the preservation of daily functions, such as eating, verbal and nonverbal communications, and the prevention of infectious diseases[3].

PRETREATMENT DENTAL CARE

While the necessity of dental clearance is debatable, assessment, treatment, and prevention of any preexisting pathological condition make up an important aspect of the overall treatment outcome in the cancer patient. While priority is given to the matter at hand, that is cancer, administering oral care in preparation for what is to come must be part of the multidisciplinary care given to the pretreatment patient. It is the ethical and medical/legal responsibility of all health care providers involved, including practitioners in the field of dentistry, to ensure that the oral health status of patients about to undergo cancer treatment is thoroughly evaluated and concerns addressed prior to the initiation of cancer therapies.

The National Institute of Dental and Craniofacial Research has developed guidelines for the provision of oral care to patients with cancer[1]. Suggested is that patients schedule a dental visit prior to beginning cancer treatment. Although there is no universally accepted pre-cancer dental protocol at this time, the dental team's involvement from early in the process may reduce the risk of oral complications in patients with poor oral health. Your cancer care team must include a dentist.

The pretreatment dental examination and visit enables the dental team to assess the status of the mouth and decide whether care should be initiated to rid the oral cavity of any acute and potentially troublesome infections, inflammation, bleeding, dental cavities, and gum related sores or lesions. The idea is to develop a comprehensive oral care plan designed to eliminate potential sites of infection that could produce complications during cancer treatment. Specific areas to address are the following:

- Necrotic (Dead) Teeth
- Mucosal (Soft Tissue Lining the Inside of the Mouth) Lesions
- Dental Cavities
- Periodontal (Gum) Disease
- Ill-Fitting Dentures or Partials
- Ill-Fitting Orthodontic Appliances
- Temporomandibular (TMJ/TMD) Malfunction
- Unsalvageable Teeth Needing Extraction
- Xerostomia (Dry Mouth)

When possible, this pre-treatment evaluation to the dentist should take place as far in advance as possible (at least one month) before the start of cancer treatment. Patients requiring oral surgery or teeth extractions must allow at least two weeks of healing before cancer treatment begins. A medical consultation should be completed before initiating any invasive procedures and collabora-tive, multidisciplinary treatment strategy created among everyone involved in the cancer care of these patients. Specifically, the primary care physician, the oncologist, the oral and maxillofacial surgeon, and the dentist together must plan and sequence the treatment involving what is to be accomplished in the oral cavity before, during, and after cancer treatment.

A comprehensive oral examination prior to initiating cancer treatment must include discussion of:

- Oral hygiene counseling focused on implementing strategies meant to reduce the oral bacterial count to a minimum while stressing specific home care instructions associated with brushing, flossing, and the use of antibacterial mouth rinses
- Tobacco cessation counseling
- Alcohol consumption cessation
- Nutritional counseling involving taking the necessary vitamins and maintaining a well-balanced diet, minimizing sharp, acidic, spicy, crunchy, and abrasive foods
- Early detection of mouth sores and lesions
- Counseling on temporary adverse effects of chemotherapy, such as neuropathy, numbness, tingling, pain, muscle weakness, or even swelling
- The use of 5000ppm fluoride applications using custom made delivery trays for the mouth
- The use of gels or topical ointments meant to soothe oral sores or lesions resulting from chemotherapy

The recommendations for pre-treatment preparations may be modified or customized to each patient as determined by the specific course of cancer treatment, the dosing of medications involved, and the location of any targeted therapeutics. Careful discussion and planning is imperative to prepare the person as a whole. Focusing on the prevention of complications during and after treatment cancer can most surely ease unexpected incidents of infection, pain, and suffering. See Table 1 below for specific guidelines on oral hygiene care for patients before beginning cancer treatment[1].

TABLE 1
Oral Hygiene Care For Patients Before Beginning Cancer Care Treatment
• Plaque removal is performed with an extra-soft nylon bristle toothbrush and gentle flossing so as not to cause trauma.
• Recommend products that are easy to grasp and manipulate (floss handle, power toothbrushes).
• Prescribe a 5000-ppm fluoride toothpaste/gel to reduce the risk of dental caries.
• Recommend products for topical management of xerostomia and oral lesions.
Specific Mucositis/Stomatitis Guidelines
• Suggest patients suck on ice chips for 30 minutes before and during chemotherapy to keep the oral cavity moist.
• Recommend patients rinse with an alkaline saline mouth rinse that includes ½ teaspoon of baking soda and ½ teaspoon of salt in 16 ounces of water. Patients should rinse at least five times per day.

In summary, a thorough head and neck evaluation, an oral hard and soft tissue examination, together with the associated intraoral radiographs are all essential parts of the initial dental visit for cancer patients. The goal is to remove and document all preexisting pathological conditions such as gum and root pathology, residual cysts, and impacted or partially erupted teeth. Through consultation with the patient's primary care and oncology physicians, oral surgery, intermediate or definitive restorations, and oral hygiene procedures may be performed safely, optimizing the patient's oral environment for minimally predictable complications.

ORAL COMPLICATIONS OF CANCER THERAPY

Oral complications are common in cancer patients. Preventing and controlling these adverse effects can help the patient continue cancer treatment and have a better quality of life. Patients receiving treatments should have their care planned by a team of doctors and specialists which include the dentist and his or her support team.

Complications are new medical problems that occur during or after a disease, procedure, or treatment that makes recovery harder. The complications may be side effects of the disease or treatment, or they may have other causes. Oral complications affect the mouth and can result in both physical trauma, an imbalance in the normal oral flora (bacterium) of the mouth, or both.

Cancer patients can have an elevated risk of oral complications for multiple reasons. Some of these may include, but are not limited to, the following:

- Chemotherapy and radiotherapy slow or stop the growth of new cells. These treatments slow or stop the growth of fast growing cells, such as cancer cells. Normal cells in the mouth also grow quickly, so anticancer treatments can stop them from growing, too. This slows down the ability of oral tissue to repair itself by making new cells.
- Radiotherapy may directly damage and breakdown oral tissue, salivary glands, and bone.
- Chemotherapy and radiotherapy upset the healthy balance of bacteria in the mouth.
- These changes may lead to mouth sores, infections, and tooth decay.

Complications And Management of Chemotherapy

Chemotherapeutic agents can damage not only the malignant cells but also the normal tissue in the patients' body. The level of toxicity greatly depends on the overall immune status of the patient prior to and during chemotherapy. In many patients, these drugs can cause several oral complications. See the Table 2 below for a list of the most common adverse effects. These include, but may not be limited to, the following conditions.

TABLE 2

Oral Complications Related to Chemotherapy

- Mucositis
- Pain
- Stomatitis
- Hemorrhage
- Xerostomia
- Neurological Issues
- Nutritional Deficiencies (Due to Inability to Eat Properly
- Fungal Infections (Candidiasis)
- Viral Infections (Herpes Simplex Virus-HSV)
- Gingival Bleeding
- Periodontal (Gum) Infection
- Taste Changes (Dysgeusia)
- Difficulty Swallowing (Dysphagia)
- Abnormal Sensations (Dysesthesia)
- Dehydration (Not Getting Enough Water Due to Inability to Drink)

Additionally, chemotherapy can decrease platelet numbers, which can increase bleeding and reduce clotting time. Furthermore, chemotherapy can lower white blood cell counts and increase the risk of infection. Blood work should be conducted 24 hours before dental treatment, assuming dental care is needed or is scheduled during chemotherapeutic care, to determine whether the patient's platelet count, clotting factors, and absolute neutrophil count are sufficient to prevent hemorrhage and infection. Treatment may need to be postponed if the platelet count is less than $50,000/mm^3$, abnormal clotting factors are present, and/or absolute neutrophil count is less than $1000/mm^3$. [1]

ORAL MUCOSITIS

Oral mucositis is the inflammation of the oral mucosa (tissue lining the inside of the mouth) resulting from chemotherapy drugs, and typically manifests as erythema (redness) or ulcerations. It presents in approximately 40% of patients receiving chemotherapy, some of which requiring medical intervention and a modification of the cyto-toxic cancer therapy. Oral mucositis usually begins seven to fourteen days after initiation of chemotherapy and remains for approximately two weeks after the regimen is complete. It often presents on the soft palate, the inner lining of the cheeks, floor of the mouth, and throat[1]. Depending on the specific class of chemotherapy drug, the mucositis may present acutely, and with or without ulcerations. Chemotherapy usually causes "acute" (transient) complications that heal after treatment ends.

Being that oral mucositis is the most common oral complication associated with chemotherapy, some therapeutic options are present here. Although not specific to mucositis, the cancer patient may find them useful in ameliorating some of the more generally painful complications mentioned above. Presently, there is no medication proven to be able to successfully eliminate mucositis[3]. However, painful symptoms can still be managed, and oral discomfort allevi-ated, to improve the patient's quality of life. The medical-dental team should be able to manage pain and encourage eating. Below, indica-tions useful for managing acute mucositis are presented. Specific instructions and indications should be discussed with the cancer care team before initiating any form of medication or application, making sure everyone involved in the care plan agrees with the prescribed care plan.

- Use of an oral solution mixture known as "**MAGIC MOUTHWASH**", composed of diphenhydramine, viscous lidocaine, bismuth, subsalicylate, and corticosteroids. It relieves acute pain and reduces inflammation, making oral consumption of food and drink much easier. The local compounding pharmacy will formulate the custom rinse according to the dentist's prescription.
- Potent **analgesic medications** (opioids) for high-grade mucositis can be made available as needed. Care should be taken to discuss analgesic selection with the whole

medical team to alleviate additional hardship on the systemic organs, such as the liver and kidney. These organs are sustaining great metabolic pressure as they work to filter and metabolize the already potent chemotherapeutic cocktails given to the cancer patient during this time.

- **Oral cryotherapy** (application of ice chips to the mouth every 30 minutes constricts blood vessels to the mucosal lining, thereby reducing the release of chemotherapeutic agents to the mucosal tissues).
- **Lower Level Laser Therapy (LLLT)** may reduce the rates of severe grade mucositis.
- Formulations containing the amino acid **L-Glutamine** and the hormone **Leptin** have shown to have a positive impact on the development of mucositis.
- Make sure to consume bland, soft, and less acidic and spicy foods during this time to minimize discomfort and introduction of new mouth sores and lesions.

ORAL INFECTIONS

Because of cancer treatments and a suppressed immune system, opportunistic bacterial, fungal, and viral infections may ensue in patients undergoing cancer therapy.

BACTERIAL INFECTIONS

Immunosuppression may cause certain bacteria in the normal oral flora to become pathogenic. Given the patient's condition, meticulous oral hygiene and the use of a prescription grade antimicrobial mouthwash containing **chlorhexidine 0.12%** is paramount. Bacteria may be removed from the teeth by using a soft bristled brush and floss at least three times per day. Acute infections localized to the oral mucosa could be treated with penicillin (barring any allergies) and metronidazole.

CANDIDIASIS INFECTIONS

The prevalence of oral fungal infections from all forms of cancer treatment is significant[3]. Use of antifungal agents, as prescribed by the patient's dentist, will assist in morbidity reduction and systemic infection prevention. Both topical and systemic forms of antifungal medications are available to the patient. Specific indications should be determined on a case by case basis and properly planned by all involved in the patient's care. As described previously, careful planning is indicated with prescribing systemic medications during this time to minimize further hardship on the filtering and metabolizing organs already in high demand (liver and kidney). Specific medications used for fungal infections, such as candidiasis, are listed below.

- Topical Antifungal Agents
- Clotrimazole Troches/Nystatin Pastilles (Mild Candidiasis)
- Nystatin Rinses
- Systemic Antifungal Agents (Specific Medications to Be Prescribed by The Treating Cancer Team)

VIRAL INFECTIONS

Herpes Simplex Virus (HSV) is prevalent in immunocompromised patients, reaching a prevalence of 40%[3]. Use of antivirals, both prophylactically and through IV (Intravenous) administration, has been shown to prevent and treat HSV. Further and more specific discussion should be had between the patient and the cancer team when deciding which of the available agents to prescribe. Two of the most commonly used antiviral medications are listed below.

- Acyclovir (Zovirax)
- Valacyclovir (Valtrex)

XEROSTOMIA (DRY MOUTH)

Cancer therapy may result in dry mouth and hyposalivation, resulting in further complications such as increased risk for dental cavities and loss of taste. Recommendations described below aim to keep the mouth as moist as possible while stimulating salivary flow.

- Take Frequent Sips of Water (Every 10 Minutes)
- Melt Ice Chips in Mouth for Comfort (Every 30 Minutes)
- Use Artificial Saliva Spray (**Xeratin, Moi-Stir, Salivart, Xero-Lube, Saliva Orthana**)
- Use Moisturizing Gel (**Biotene®, Oral Balance**)
- Lubricate Lips with Petroleum Jelly or A Lanolin-Containing Preparation (**bioXtra**)
- Discontinue Coffee, Tea, Soft Drinks with Caffeine
- Use Alcohol-Free Mouth Rinses (**bioXtra, Biotene®, Oral Seven**)
- Use Saliva Stimulating Tablets (SST) and Pilocarpine (**Salagen**) Medications to Increase Salivary Flow
- Use **Sorbitol** or **Xylitol-Based Chewing Gum** for Salivary Flow Stimulation and Caries Prevention

DYSGEUSIA (TASTE CHANGES)

About 50% to 70% of patients receiving chemotherapy, radiotherapy, or both will suffer from a distorted or an impaired ability to taste, contributing to eventual weight loss and nutritional imbalances. Varying degrees of saliva gland disruption and damage may ensue from low to high doses of chemotherapeutic agents and irradiation. Whether the adverse effects are transient or chronic will be determined by the extent of therapy and on the specific location the targeted treatment is aimed at. Several studies have suggested the following with attempts to ameliorate this oral complication.

- Zinc Supplementation May Regulate Taste Bud Pores
- Vitamin D Supplementation
- Nutritional Counseling

- Drinking Plenty of Fluids During Administration of Cytotoxic Medications
- Chewing Food Slowly and Thoroughly to Release More Flavors and Stimulate Saliva Production
- Switching Foods During Meals to Prevent Adaptation of Taste Receptors
- Maintaining A Balanced Diet

A helpful guide to understanding what to ask and how to manage oral health during chemotherapy can be reviewed in Table 3 below[1].

TABLE 3
Patient information that may be helpful to have prior to the pretreatment dental visit:
• What is my complete blood count, including absolute neutrophil and platelet counts?
• If an invasive dental procedure is necessary, do I have adequate clotting factors present?
• What is the scheduled sequence of treatment so that safe dental care can be planned?
• Is radiation therapy also planned?
What the patient should expect during oral assessments:
• Evaluation of soft tissues for inflammation and infection
• Evaluation of plaque levels and presence of dental caries
• Management of oral lesions/mucositis
• Management of xerostomia
• Education about the importance of oral health
• Nutritional Counseling
• Assessment of inflammation and soreness of mucous membranes
Diet and Lifestyle Considerations:
• Consume soft, moist foods
• Consume liquids such as broth, yogurt, or other liquids if swallowing is difficult
• Use of mild-flavored toothpastes (non-mint)
• Avoid spicy, acidic, hard/sharp (chips, toast crusts), and hot foods and beverages
• Avoid tobacco and alcohol consumption
Mucosal Coating Agents:
• Antacid Solutions
• Kaolin Solutions
• Saliva Substitutes
• Topical Anesthetics
• Cellulose Film-Forming Agents

Complications and Management of Radiotherapy

As in chemotherapy, orofacial tissues that may be inflamed by radiotherapy to the proximal anatomy include salivary glands, taste buds, mucous membranes, bone and teeth, the temporomandibular join (TMJ), and related musculatures. Acute effects usually develop early in the radiation treatment period and persist for 2-3 weeks after its completion. Late or chronic effects may arise at any time after completion of treatment, ranging from weeks to years. Although, currently, there is scant evidence regarding oral complications of breast irradiation, several of the adverse effects are like those resulting from chemotherapy. The more common issues to be concerned about are listed below in TABLE 4.

TABLE 4
Oral Complications Related to Radiotherapy
• Xerostomia (Dry Mouth)
• Oral Discomfort and Pain
• Oral Infections
• Difficulties in Speech, Chewing, And Swallowing
• Increased Risk of Dental Caries
• Radiation-Induced Mucositis
• Taste Loss (Dysgeusia)
• Inability to Swallow Well (Dysphagia)
• Osteoradionecrosis (Inability for Bone to Repair Itself or Tolerate Trauma Due to Bone and Blood Cell Damage)

It is now widely accepted that, through the generation of free radicals, ionizing radiation can cause alteration of the vascular elements in the bone within the irradiated fields[3]. The result is an area described as one possessing minimal ability to withstand trauma, or to be repaired. Procedures such as dental extractions, dental implant placement, or other forms of jaw surgery involving bone injury may pose a risk for the cancer patient receiving significant doses of radiation to the head, neck, or jaw area. This condition, known as osteoradionecrosis, is in fact not a common complication of radiotherapy[3]. Despite this fact, discussion on how to prevent such a complication should still be a key component of the cancer care plan considered during the pretreatment dental visit. Together with the primary care and oncology physicians, the dentist's responsibility is to educate the patient on this risk and to thoroughly evaluate the mouth for potential sites of current or future infection related to bone pathology or hopeless teeth in need of immediate care or extraction.

COMPLICATIONS AND MANAGEMENT OF ANTIESTROGEN THERAPY

Current adjuvant treatment modalities for breast cancer that express the estrogen receptor or progesterone receptor include anti-estrogen therapies, tamoxifen and aromatase inhibitors. Bone, including the jaw, is an endocrine sensitive organ, as are other oral structures. Although periodontal diseases, alveolar bone density, tooth loss, and conditions of the soft tissues of the mouth have all been associated with menopausal status supporting the hypothesis that they can all be negatively affected by anti-estrogen therapy, the impact of adjunctive endocrine breast cancer therapy on the oral health of post-menopausal women is undefined. The structures of the oral cavity are influenced by estrogen; therefore, anti-estrogen therapies may carry the risk of oral toxicities.

The decrease in estrogen levels among post-menopausal women has been associated with reduced salivary flow. Recently, aromatase inhibitors, which severely diminish estrogen levels, have been shown to impact periodontal health and increase levels of xerostomia in breast cancer patients. Decreased salivary flow can result in gingival bleeding and dental caries and may be responsible for an increased prevalence of oral dysesthesia (abnormal sensation) and alterations in taste sensation. Additionally, women using anti-estrogen therapies may experience greater levels of depression, musculoskeletal symptoms and fatigue, impacting their ability to achieve optimal oral health[1].

Dental professionals and patients alike should be aware of the potential changes in periodontal tissues. The risk of xerostomia and the psychological implications associated with patients undergoing anti-estrogen therapies should be closely monitored to address these issues and counsel the patient during this time. Table 5 below summarizes the complications associated with anti-estrogen therapy for the breast cancer patient.

TABLE 5
Oral Complications Related to Anti-Estrogen Therapy
• Reduced Salivary Flow
• Affect Periodontal Health
• Increase Levels of Xerostomia
• Gingival Bleeding
• Dental Caries
• Oral Dysesthesia (Abnormal Sensation)
• Dysgeusia (Altered Taste Sensation)
• Increased Levels of Depression
• Musculoskeletal Symptoms
• Fatigue
• Compromised Oral Health

Complications and Management of Bisphosphonate Therapy

Bisphosphonates are a class of drugs that are used to prevent bone loss demineralization (weakening or destruction). Some of these drugs can be taken by mouth, while others must be given intravenously at a hospital or clinic. Examples include drugs such as Actonel, Zometa, Fosamax, and Boniva.

While the most common indication for oral Bisphosphonates is to treat osteoporosis, indications for intravenous (IV) Bisphosphonates include treatment and management of cancer-related conditions including hypercalcemia of malignancy, skeletal related events associated with bone metastases in the context of solid tumors such as breast cancer, prostate cancer and lung cancer, and management of lesions in the setting of multiple myeloma.

The clinical efficacy of IV Bisphosphonates for the treatment of bone metastasis and hypercalcemia as related to breast cancer is well established. As synthetic analogs of naturally occurring pyrophosphates, they inhibit bone resorption and therefore improve bone mineral density by decreasing bone turn over. For this reason, they have a wide application in oral diseases, such as oral cancer, breast cancer, osteogenesis imperfect, fibrous dysplasia, hypercalcemia, etc. In cases of breast cancer metastasis to bone, the use of IV Bisphosphonates helps to inhibit osteoclastic-mediated (bone destroying) bone resorption (destruction), allowing these medications to act as "bone protective agents".

Although highly efficacious in the treatment of bone metastasis as related to breast cancer, long term use of IV Bisphosphonates is associated with its own adverse effects. Osteonecrosis of the jaws is a major complication associated with its use. The synergistic effect of the combination of chemotherapy, Bisphosphonate-induced cellular stress due to long term use, cancer related co-morbid factors, uncoupling of osteoblast-osteoclast equilibrium, reduced vasculature, bone microfractures, and tracking of oral microbes through the periodontium may act in concert to produce a "bandwagon" effect that raises disease burden and lower susceptibilities threshold in favor of Bisphosphonate-related Osteonecrosis of the Jaw (BONJ)[6].

Breast cancer patients may find themselves at a higher risk for Bisphosphonate-related osteonecrosis of the jaw (BONJ). As described previously, osteonecrosis is a problem with bone healing that can occur when damage is done to osteocytes (bone cells); furthermore, impairment to the bone's blood supply prevents adequate jaw bone repair after dental surgery, trauma, or extraction of teeth.

It is of the utmost importance for the breast cancer patient receiving IV Bisphosphonates to make certain that therapy management strategies are discussed and thoroughly communicated among the dental and medical professionals comprising the cancer care team.

Oral and Maxillofacial surgeons first recognized and reported cases of non-healing exposed bone in the maxillofacial region in patients treated with IV Bisphosphonates. Moreover, epidemiologic studies have established a compelling association between IV Bisphosphonates and BONJ in the setting of malignant disease[5].

Patients may be considered to have **BRONJ** if all the following three characteristics are present[5].

- Current or Previous Treatment with A Bisphosphonate
- Exposed Bone in The Maxillofacial Region That Persisted for More Than Eight Weeks
- No History of Radiation Therapy to The Jaws

DENTAL IMPLICATIONS OF BISPHOSPHONATE THERAPY

Most reported cases of BONJ have been diagnosed after dental procedures such as tooth extraction. Less commonly, BONJ appears to occur spontaneously in patients taking these drugs[6]. The dentist must know the patient's history and susceptibility to oral disease. And, the patient must relay the use of oral or IV Bisphosphonates to the dentist of record. Together, the cancer care team can provide guidance and recommendations intended to reduce the incidence of oral complications during cancer treatment.

BONJ can occur spontaneously, owing to dental disease or secondary to dental therapy. If possible, bisphosphonate therapy should be delayed when dental health is sub-optimal. Invasive dental procedures should be completed; non-restorable teeth with poor prognosis should be extracted. Patients are still instructed to keep taking the bisphosphonates for an extended amount of time, since the benefits of these are well established. Some of the oral diseases such as periapical (root surrounding tissues) pathoses, sinus tracts, pus-containing abscesses which involve the bone, may cause osteonecrosis by themselves. Such cases should be treated immediately[6].

Because evidence also supports an infectious and possibly immunologic underlying cause for BONJ, before starting Bisphosphonate therapy, the patient should be referred for a thorough dental evaluation to identify and treat any potential sources of infection. The dentist should provide oral hygiene instructions and ensure dental prophylaxis is done. Consultation with an oral surgeon or dentist familiar with cancer care management is imperative. Patients already on Bisphosphonates who are receiving dental treatment have been found to be at risk of experiencing delayed healing from tooth extractions and spontaneous soft-tissue breakdown leading to intra-oral bone exposure[6]. Placing the patient on a broad-spectrum antibi-otic prior to beginning a dental procedure may be considered. Close collaboration with the patient's oncologist is highly recommended when considering the administration of antibiotics or the adjustment of cancer treatment medications. Patients experiencing early signs of asymptomatic oral disease while on Bisphosphonates should be placed on antimicrobial rinses containing 0.12% chlorhexidine, while patients experiencing exposed bone associated with pain may benefit from a combination of 0.12% chlorhexidine rinse and systemic antibi-otics based on culture and sensitivity tests.

Regarding dental implantology, the patient taking IV Bisphospho-nates should not consider the placement of dental implants during this time. Because the surgery involves bone injury and manipula-tion, careful consideration must be had. Plans should be made for dental implant placement after the cancer therapy has ceased and sufficient time has passed since the IV Bisphosphonates were discon-tinued. Although oral Bisphosphonates do not seem to pose the same risk if the patient has been taking them for less than three years, careful discussion with the primary care physician and oncologist is recommended prior to initiating any type of invasive dental proce-dure involving surgery or bone injury. Maintenance of existing implants should follow accepted mechanical and pharmaceutical methods to prevent peri-implantitis (inflammation/infection of the tissues surrounding the implant), with regular monitoring of the patient. In short, long term Bisphosphonate use, or current adminis-tration of IV Bisphosphonates, should be treated with caution.

Barring any kind of surgically invasive procedures, all routine restorative procedures, including non-surgical endodontic and prosthodontic care, can be carried out. No evidence suggests the development of BONJ as related to routine dentistry. Patients wearing removable dentures or partials should be cautioned against the use of ill-fitting appliances that may be causing friction, mucosal trauma, or mouth sores, especially along the lower jaw bone, or mandible. If BONJ has already developed in this patient, dental management will depend on the severity of the lesion. In such patients, the goal would be to eliminate pain, controlling hard and soft tissue infections, and minimizing the progression of osteonecrosis[6]. Consultation with the oncologist is recommended should the dentist consider the discontinuation of the Bisphosphonate.

Routine dental treatment generally should not be modified solely based on oral Bisphosphonate therapy; a thorough medical history is essential. Whether oral or IV Bisphosphonates are involved, the dentist and physician managing patient must adopt an interdisciplinary approach that will result in the formulation of an effective patient-specific management protocol. The dentist's role as part of the medical treatment team is particularly important to enhancing the quality of life for these often very ill patients. Close follow-up every three to four months is imperative to track the progress of the disease and to be on the lookout for any side effects that may arise from Bisphosphonate therapy[6].

POST CANCER TREATMENT ORAL CARE

Now that much discussion has been had about how to prepare the oral environment for cancer therapy and later manage the intraoral complications that may arise from aggressive administration of drugs and modalities, we should now briefly remind the cancer patient that after-cancer treatment care is just as important to maintaining a good quality of life. Post cancer care of the mouth should play as important a role in the patient's self-care as any other wellness related recommendation given by the cancer care team. The oral cavity is often the first view into what is happening systemically. Medical conditions such as cardiovascular disease, diabetes, and inflammatory diseases are oftentimes related to what is also present in the oral cavity.

Studies have shown that the inflammatory factors and bacterial flora associated with periodontal disease are similar, if not identical, to those found in cardiovascular disease. Furthermore, certain diseases such as diabetes have been shown to worsen as the periodontal health of the patient deteriorates; the opposite is also true. Uncontrolled diabetes is known to negatively affect the healing capacity and stability of periodontal disease.

The mouth is connected to the rest of the body. It is imperative for patients and health professionals alike to recognize and understand the implications associated with this fact. It is the responsibility of the patient to make sure he or she is compliant with maintaining regular dental visits to detect early signs of instability or imbalance to the wellness of the oral cavity. Because the mouth mirrors what may be happening systemically, the opposite is also true. Systemic imbalance could be detected orally and recognized initially by the vigilant and thorough dental physician.

One's nutrition plays a vital role in maintaining optimal oral health. Consumption of foods and beverages high is sugar and acidic content contributes to a higher incidence of decay (dental cavities) and tooth sensitivity, especially in those patients having undergone higher doses of radiotherapy, resulting in chronic xerostomia (dry mouth). These patients will forever need to protect their dentition from enamel erosion, dental decay, tooth sensitivity, and restorative breakdown. Generally speaking, the human microbiome (collection of organisms living inside the human body) is a collection of microbes, which include bacteria, viruses, and fungi that exist in and on our bodies-and in our environment. Some of these microbes work in sync with our bodies and others are harmful to the human and are often disease causing. Our bodies are usually pretty good at keeping things in balance, and that balance of microbes helps lead to health. Having a balance between the beneficial bugs and those more prone to cause harm leads to a healthy and calm state. But, when our bodies' microbes are out of balance, disease occurs. And that is where the association with cancer may come in. Studies are currently underway to better understand the relationship between a microbiome imbalance and the development of our immune system, and how this may affect the incidence of cancer. Certain microorganisms are known to cause cancer if allowed to influence cellular changes within the body. One factor here is to maintain a well-balanced diet that can positively nurture the immune system. In doing so, the body is better able to combat potential microbial imbalance and maybe even respond better to cancer therapies that would otherwise not be as successful.

Now that a brief discussion shed light on the importance of oral and whole person balance, the cancer patient needs to also plan to restore failed dental treatment or replace missing teeth, either present before cancer care or existing now because of it. Discussion with the dentist should be had to determine the best options available to the patient's specific needs. Restoratively speaking, definitive restoration of dental decay, periodontal disease, and chronic infection can now be planned in conjunction with a medical clearance from the oncologist and primary care physician. From a structural and cosmetic stand point, various dental restorative options are available for discussion. These may include, but are not limited to:

- Tooth Colored Fillings
- Teeth Whitening
- Porcelain Crowns and Veneers
- Fixed Porcelain Bridges to Replace Missing Teeth
- Fixed Single or Multiple Dental Implants to Replace One Or More Teeth
- Fixed Implant Supported Dentures
- Fixed Implant Supported Teeth in A Day Restorations
- Traditional Removable Full or Partial Dentures (Not Recommended as Definitive Restorations)

Although comprehensive, the list above does not describe all scenarios or treatment modalities available today. Patient-specific options would be determined based on an oral assessment, condition of the oral cavity, patient desires and limitations, patient compliance, medical history and status, and other factors. To further your long-term care, patients should continue to use products designed to remineralize the teeth, reduce the risk of dental caries, reduce tooth sensitivity, eliminate tissue inflammation, moisten the mouth, and freshen the breath. The same products described in previous sections may continue to be used after cancer care, and as needed. Together with a well-balanced diet and regular dental examinations, optimal oral health can be maintained.

Patients must find educated, caring, dedicated, and compassionate dentists that are willing and able to integrate medicine into their delivery of care. As I stated previously, the mouth does not stand alone; it is a vital and living component of our body. It houses blood, nerve, and lymphatic systems that connect to the rest of the body. Take care of it and learn how to use it as mirror into the rest of YOU.

In conclusion, I would like to commend you on your commitment to learn, to better understand, and to actively engage in your cancer care. Your courage will help you along the way. Successful treatment CANNOT happen without a positive and enduring spirit. I wish you health, happiness, and hope for better days ahead. Thank you for allowing me to share in this journey with you. It has been my privilege to do so.

Refrerences

1. Taichman LS, Tindle D. Oral Health Maintenance For Patients With Breast Cancer. The Journal Of Multidisciplinary Care; Decisions In Dentistry: 2016 January
2. Taichman LS, Gomez G, Inglehart Mr. Oral Health-Related Complications Of Breast Cancer Treatment: Assessing Dental Hygienists' Knowledge and Professional

Practice. Journal of Dental Hygiene: JDH. 2015; 89 (Supp 12):22-37.

3. Wong, Hai (2014). Oral Complications and Management Strategies for Patients Undergoing Cancer Therapy. The Scientific World Journal. 2014.581795.10.1155/2014 1581795.

4. Breast Cancer Research and Treatment Journal. US National Library of Medicine.

5. American Association of Oral and Maxillofacial Surgeons Position Paper on Bisphosphonate-Related Osteonecrosis of the Jaws. Advisory Task Force on Bisphosphonate-Related Osteonecrosis of the Jaws. J Oral and Maxillofacial Surgery 65: 2007.

6. JIOH Volume 4; Issue 2: May-Aug 2012 www.ispcd.org J. Int Oral Health 2012 Bisphosphonate in Oral Diseases; Updates of Its Implications in Dental Management. Jayalakshmi K Rovikumar HJaya Naidu Archana Patil

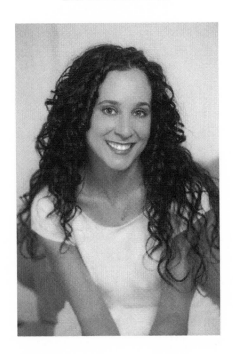

Rita Dargham, D.M.D

Recognized as one of South Florida's leading family cosmetic and restorative dentists, Dr. Rita Dargham has over a decade of experience in the art and science of creating healthy and beautiful smiles. Dr. Dargham completed her undergraduate studies at the University of Miami where she earned a Bachelor of Science in Biology, later proceeding to the University of Florida where she graduated with honors, earning her Doctorate in Medical Dentistry in May of 1997. Furthering her studies, she completed her post-graduate training at the Miami Veterans Administration Hospital, concentrating on dental implant and reconstructive dentistry.

Respected for her expertise in Smile Reconstruction and Enhancement, Dr. Dargham's philosophy is centered in achieving the balance between health and natural beauty when designing her patients' smile image. Customized technology, utilizing both traditional and digital techniques, enables the creation of naturally appearing porcelain veneers, crowns, bondings, tooth-colored fillings, and dental implants in the design of single tooth or full mouth restorations. Dedication to excellence has afforded Dr. Dargham the ability to provide her patients with long-lasting dentistry they would be proud to call their own for many years to come. Whether with Invisalign orthodontics, teeth whitening, or dental dermal fillers and Botox, Dr. Dargham's experience has enabled beautiful and healthy smiles.

Dr. Dargham is an active member of numerous well-respected dental organizations and educational institutes that serve to continuously enhance her ability to provide her patients with successful treatment in all facets of dentistry. She serves as a participant in the Florida Dental Association, the American Dental Association, the American Academy of Cosmetic Dentistry, the LD Pankey Institute, and the Seattle Study Club Organization, among others.

Through Operation Smile, a nonprofit medical organization, Dr. Dargham has discovered an invaluable way to see the world while simultaneously donating her time and expertise to treat children and young adults suffering from the ill-effects of a congenital defect known as cleft lip and palate. While visiting numerous underdeveloped countries, she has offered education, treatment and support to these underprivileged societies. The experience of watching a child enjoy the new-found ability to function and smile has served as a life-altering and rewarding gift.

Dr. Dargham continues to enjoy what has become a wonderful journey mastering the Art of Designing Beautiful and Healthy Smiles. The diversity in cultures she has had the pleasure of experiencing within her family of patients has allowed her to learn and appreciate the vast array of attributes that bring a smile to people from all walks of life.

14

NUTRITION: A HIGHER LEVEL OF WELLBEING

SABRINA HERNANDEZ-CANO, RDN, CDE, NC

"Health is a state of complete harmony of the body, mind and spirit. When one is free from physical disabilities and mental distractions, the gates of the soul open."

— B.K.S. IYENGAR

Anyone can be diagnosed with breast cancer even without having obvious risk factors. One in eight women will develop breast cancer in their lifetime. There have been many who were shocked when test results revealed there was a lump in their breast. I have friends, cousins, aunts, colleagues, clients and even my own mother –who were taken by surprise by news of this health crisis. They felt their healthy lifestyle, eating well etc. would shelter them from this diagnosis. That is why I believe there is so much frustration with this diagnosis. We do the best we can with the food we eat, our exercise routine and our environment. However, there are no guarantees that will equal a disease-free life and we would do well to remember that health is a journey, not a destination. As such, we need to remain vigilant and be aware of risk factors, then aim to reduce them.

My goal in this chapter on nutrition is to share my years of experience and knowledge and offer what I have gathered from nature, science, and survivors so that we may obtain a higher level of wellness through proper nutrition. If we must face a breast cancer diagnosis, let us do so with a stronger mind and body to help us heal and recover with the optimum cellular strength that the right nutrition provides.

I am a strong believer in proper nourishment. It starts when we choose natural foods, activate our bodies, and positively feed our mind and spirit to the best of our ability. Wellness is an interior mirror looking from the outside in and reflecting from the inside out. Poor nutrition, stress, a sedentary lifestyle, and a toxic environment are a pretty good recipe for most types of cancers.

We need to ask ourselves some basic yet important questions. Are we choosing chemical-laden, artificial junk food? Do we neglect our basic need for the proper amount of water? Do we lack movement and become so rigid and tight that our bodies just don't flow? Do we know the distribution of our weight so we know just how much fat mass or muscle mass we carry? Do we give into excess sugar and alcohol because we buy into sweet and sexy marketing?

It is time for us to become aware and to question why it is that in our great nation, losing weight has become a 50 billion dollar industry. If we continue to buy junk food, manufacturers will continue to package it nicely for us. Our future generations may find themselves eating from boxes and wrappers filled with processed and non-nutritious, difficult-to-pronounce mystery ingredients that may not even classify as food. I invite you to commit to a higher level of wellbeing and to switch to natural foods and properly nourish our physical, emotional, intellectual, social and spiritual being. Strength, flexibility and endurance are a reflection of wellness. This wellness will lead to mental focus, clarity and longevity.

My experience as an overweight child inspired me to change and improve my nutrition. The struggle to fit in, and the name calling I experienced was so strong that I found myself making better food choices, eating smaller portions, and dancing my way into a career that if given the chance I would choose all over again. Today, my inspiration comes from the opportunity I have to see my clients transform, eat right and find enjoyable ways to move their bodies every day.

Prevention is Paramount

Staying informed of the latest research is the key to prevention and care. Science, research and technology have had a huge impact on the number of lives saved and the quality of those lives has improved as well. While there are certain habits and practices we know for certain can lower risk factors there are other that are still not so clear. However, one thing is absolutely indisputable: weight matters. Scientists are telling us that gaining weight as we age increases the risk of post-menopausal breast cancer. A combination of excess weight and higher levels of estrogen and insulin may also be a detrimental triangle.

Avoiding obesity, which is correlated with high-circulating insulin levels, is crucial in preventing breast and other cancers. Post-menopausal women do not produce estrogen. Their fat cells become responsible for making estrogen; therefore, the more fat cells in the body, the higher the amount of estrogen as estradiol in their blood, which increases risk.

Overwhelming evidence supported by in-vitro, animal, and epidemiologic studies suggest that lifestyle and diet influence cancer initiation, promotion, and progression. Currently, according to the American Cancer Society (ACS), 60-70 percent of all cancer cases are directly related to the foods we eat and the way we live. The ACS also estimates that by simply choosing a better lifestyle and getting your physician to perform a health screening could prevent half of all cancer-related deaths. This suggests we have control over our health.

It is never too early or too late to take charge of our own wellbeing and eat a healthy diet. Dietary guidelines for cancer prevention are very much like those for avoiding the risk of other health problems including heart disease, diabetes, Alzheimer's, and high blood pressure.

Despite the fact that there are over 17,500 diets in existence and a 50 billion dollar industry in weight-loss products that may or may not work to go along with them, the most scientifically convincing evidence for cancer-fighting potential proves that maintaining or achieving a healthy weight 2. Becoming physically active, exploring the power of nutritious foods, and staying nutritionally strong during the fight are our ammunition. These factors define what a promising nutritious lifestyle is all about. In this chapter, you will also find super nutritious, delicious recipes and meal plans that promote optimal health.

Weight Matters

Charts or scales alone do not determine healthy weight. Your personal healthy weight is unique to you; just as you are special in many ways, so are your height, size, and shape. This is why your genetic makeup plays a strong role. A genetic link may also exist to body fat. However, we cannot blame genes alone.

Metabolism (the rate at which your body burns energy) differs from woman to woman. Patients love it when they finally understand body composition. A machine called the Tanita Body Composition Analyzer runs a small current up one leg and down the other. There is no pain during this procedure. The patients get a readout that shows not only their weight but also their muscle and fat mass. Because muscle burns more calories than fat, it is advisable to become physically active and increase muscle mass. Healthy weight is also determined by your body mass index (BMI). This is simply your weight in relation to your height (see Chart 1) for an easy way to figure your BMI.

Simply plot your height in inches: for example, if you are five feet tall, that's sixty inches; if you are five feet, two inches tall, that's sixty-two inches. Now find your weight across and your BMI above. This tool also helps determine your risk for weight-related health problems. BMI is usually higher in women with more percentage of fat than those with higher percentage of muscle. Women with excess body fat are at greater risk for health problems including cancer. The higher the BMI is, the greater the risk for cancer. A BMI of 18.5 to 24.9 indicates a healthy weight; 25 to 30, overweight; and 30 and higher, obesity.

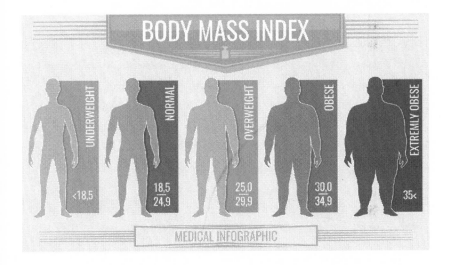

To be in a healthy weight range, aim for a BMI of 18.5 to 24. Do not forget that a healthy you can come in many different sizes and shapes. This makes you a special individual and a beautiful woman.

The most important thing about your weight is to keep it within a healthy range so you can enjoy a fuller, more productive life and reduce your risk of disease. If your BMI is above 25 or 30, there is some work to be done. Clearly, there is a link between obesity and breast cancer. The reason I know this is because at this moment there are at least 107 research-based articles on my desk tell me so.

Experts and researchers on diet and cancer prevention note that obesity (BMI 30 or above) affects hormones and hormone-related cancers. Cancer is on the rise every year and, unfortunately, so is our weight as a nation. We are facing an epidemic of obesity and we must stop it or we will continue to see more health problems in the future. Just as we fight to find a cure for breast cancer, we must use our ammunition to fight obesity.

The National Cancer Institute says obesity and inactivity may account for up to 20-30 percent of breast, colon, uterine, kidney, and esophageal cancers. It seems that obesity is a major risk factor for breast cancer in post-menopausal women, but not for premenopausal women. Studies are also suggesting that excessive body fat also decreases chances of recovery from cancer. The reason is that excess fatty tissue is a main source of circulating a hormone called estrogen in your body. And breast cancer risk is linked to how much estrogen you are exposed to during your lifetime.

A research study found that women who gained weight after their breast cancer diagnosis increased their risk of recurrence. Excess weight also increases levels of another hormone called insulin, which in turn fuels estrogen. Estrogen is linked to breast and endometrial cancers.

By now, you have seen that although research always has something new to say, many sources from all over the world say the same thing when it comes to weight. Research in achieving or maintaining a healthy weight and lowering the risk of first–time breast cancer also suggest that overweight women have an increased risk of breast cancer – especially after menopause – as compared to women at a healthy weight during this time in their lives.

In a 2005 analysis, Harvard Medical School indicated that losing five to twenty pounds may reduce your cancer risk by 10 percent. Losing more may provide more protection. No matter how much weight you need to lose, even a small loss will offer benefits. So then, how do you lose weight?

This is the fifty-billion-dollar question. First, beware: Almost all of us have contributed to this amount by buying headlines that are just too good to pass up, even if they don't make sense at all. You know, the ones that read, "Lose 10 pounds in three days."

Yeah, right, sure—only in my dreams.

It just doesn't make any scientific or mathematical sense at all. Before I even attempt to explain how to lose weight, let me remind you that I was an overweight child. Eating on smaller plates, commitment, determination, and a bit of physical activity helped me achieve a healthy weight. You can do the same.

A healthy diet requires that you eat not only the right kind of food, but also the right amount. Excess food that is more than the amount your body requires turns into excess energy or calories that get stored as fat. Since proper nutrition is one of the cornerstones for cancer prevention, let's figure out how many calories promote a healthy weight.

Even though you may need to reach weight goals, it is not advisable to lose weight during cancer treatment. During cancer therapies such as chemotherapy and radiation therapy, you need to eat to your full potential to maximize the amount of nutrients so your body can be strong to fight along with the medical treatments.

The American Cancer Society has reported that one third of cancer deaths were related to nutrition, physical inactivity, and obesity. Let's do the math. If we are going to lose or gain weight, we need to know that there are 3,500 calories in one pound of fat. The cause of being overweight is an energy imbalance: more calories consumed than used. To figure out how many calories you need, simply take your healthy weight in pounds from the BMI chart and multiply by 10 for women and 11 for men. Calories for basic needs, depending on how active you are, would be added 20 percent for light activity, 30 percent for moderate activity, and 50 percent for high activity.

For example: Required Daily Calorie Intake for a 140-Pound Woman

140x10=1,400. Add 20 percent or 280 for light activity.

1,400 +280 =1,680 calories and activity= total calories need

If your BMI is 25 or above and you need to lose weight, take your present weight and divide it by 2.2. Then multiply by 25 and subtract 500 calories to reveal the number of calories you need to eat on a daily basis to promote one pound of fat loss per week: 1,700 calories for a 200–pound woman will promote 1 pound per week weight loss, which is safe.

Although this should give you an idea of how important it is to consider calories in weight management, it is not a substitute for a consultation with a registered dietitian who can provide an individualized program.

Using medical nutrition therapy, a registered dietitian will tailor strategies to your budget, schedule, special needs, and the needs of your family. To find a registered dietitian in your area you can go to the American Dietetic Association web site at www.eatright.org.

Always consult with your physician before starting any weight–loss or physical activity program. In order to be successful in any weight–loss endeavor, you must have internal motivators – things like your good health, increased energy and stamina, self-esteem, and a commitment to yourself and your health goals. Your commitment should be for a lifetime and not just for the summer to fit into that cute bathing suit.

Ten Strategies and Ammunition for Successful Weight Loss

1. **Commit** as if you were getting married to form a good relationship with food.
2. **Forget** your total weight. Know your Fat Mass in pounds. Don't weigh yourself daily.
3. **Tweak** all your meals. That means cut the portions of the foods you choose in half.
4. **Whatever** you do, don't start a diet. Its only a few days away from ending and making you feel like a failure. Know your calorie intake and listen to your body. Eat

when you are hungry and stop eating when you are satisfied.

5. **Make** a wish list of all the foods you wish you were eating. Buy at least three every time you grocery-shop. Allow yourself pleasures in moderation and let go of toxic behaviors with food.

6. **Don't** buy anything in large quantities. Even children should get used to smaller containers and bags.

7. **Eat** several times throughout the day.

8. **Read** labels and know what they mean.

9. **Leave** emotions out. Mindfully connect to your hunger and fullness cues.

10. **Get** physical.

The Best Diet is Knowledge

- **Calories** come from carbohydrates, proteins, fats, and alcohol. Calories that come from fat and alcohol supply more calories than carbohydrates and proteins, per gram.

- **Carbohydrates** and proteins have fewer calories per gram, while fats supply nine calories, and alcohol seven calories Carbohydrates are the main energy source for the body. They are the body's basic fuel. We need them in the right quantity and of the right quality. This means choosing whole grains such as bulgur, quinoa, high–fiber cereals, and brown and wild rice. These are more nutritious because they have the bran and germ, which are rich in vitamins, minerals, fiber and phytochemicals. Go easy on refined white grains such as pasta, rice, and white bread and rolls. Avoiding them in excess is best. They do not contribute as much nutrition and increase the need for more insulin. I find this makes one hungrier and therefore more prone to overeating.

Research is now suggesting that these carbohydrates, which are low in fiber, may cause spikes in blood sugar because they are quickly converted into glucose. Whole grains are digested slowly and have a lower impact on blood sugar.

A study co-sponsored by the American Institute for Cancer Research reported that women who ate the most carbohydrates were more than twice as likely to have breast cancer as those who ate less. The lowest rates of breast cancer were in women who ate higher amounts of insoluble fiber found in whole–grain carbohydrates such as bran cereals, whole wheat bread, and vegetables. Fiber is a variety of compounds, which have different effects on the body. There are two categories of fiber, soluble and insoluble. Soluble fiber is the one that evidence suggest helps to lower cholesterol and may reduce the risk of heart disease. Soluble fiber sources include oats, oat bran, barley, beans or legumes, fruits, vegetables, and brown rice. Insoluble fiber is the one that aids in constipation when consumed with plenty of water. In one reported study in the Journal of the American Medical Association, a diet high in fiber helped in controlling weight gain and insulin levels.

I encourage my patients to consume 20-30 grams of fiber daily, and to look for good sources of fiber on the labels: 3 grams or more per serving. The research on fiber is ongoing and not yet conclusive, but researchers agree there is plenty of evidence that a diet rich in fiber based on whole grains, fruits, and vegetables may protect against many chronic diseases. This may be because fiber curbs insulin secretion and fiber-rich carbohydrates often contain anti-cancer substances.

- **Proteins:** This macronutrient earns the superlative vote for most popular; everyone wants to eat it for power and strength. It's true our bodies use protein to build and repair; however, it is important to understand that there are the same calories – 4 to be exact – per gram in both carbohydrates and proteins. Extra protein also gets stored

as fat. It is important to be mindful of portions. Choose
lean meats such as chicken, fish, shellfish and more
vegetable proteins. Good sources of vegan protein include
garbanzo beans, lentils, soybeans and edamame.
Vegetables such as peas, spinach, broccoli and brussel
sprouts also contribute protein.

- **Fats:** Research is still not yet conclusive on the association
  of eating a low-fat diet and the prevention of breast cancer.
  Some scientists are suggesting that there might be a link
  between estrogen and fat intake: When dietary fat
  increases, estrogen levels in breast tissue also go up, which
  may provoke cancer growth. What we are sure of is that
  overall food choices that are lower in fat such as fruits,
  vegetables, and whole grains do offer protection not just
  for your breasts but for your heart as well. A high–fat diet,
  especially from animal fat such as saturated fat and Trans
  fatty acids, has been linked to some types of cancers
  including breast, colon, rectum, and lung. In addition to
  aiming for a low-fat diet, it is also important to consume
  the right kind of fat.

But let's first define fat and the role it plays in our system. Fat,
according to Webster's dictionary, is fleshy, plump, oily, rich, and
resinous. Fat means so many different things to so many different
people. Most women have something to say about "fat" in their lives. I
remember Oprah Winfrey talking about it when I was a kid.

"Too much on the thighs, hips, and booty" or "too little on the
breast, legs, and ankles." Whether women struggle with obesity or
battle anorexia, fat in the last decade has become a hot topic. And
with the latest research on the overall health benefits of oils, it seems
the whole country is turning toward a positive attitude about fats.
Fats are essential to good health; they perform crucial bodily functions. No human being can live without them. Fats are like a fancy jet
plane. They transport special vitamins such as A, D, E and K, as well

as carotenoids into the bloodstream. That is why these important vitamins are called the fat-soluble vitamins. Fat also aids in the maintenance of cell membrane, structure, and function. And most importantly, it preserves one's immune system.

The kind of fat that we choose to eat can actually benefit or harm us. There are healthy and harmful fats. So let's set the record straight. You can start choosing the best oils for overall health, including breast cancer prevention.

Monounsaturated

Monounsaturated fat is called mono because there is only one hydrogen on the carbon chain. The body can process one hydrogen more easily than a chain that is fully saturated with several hydrogen. Okay, enough organic chemistry. Monounsaturated fats are liquid at room temperature and begin to solidify in the refrigerator. Monounsaturated fats such as olive, peanut, and canola (avocados and most nuts also have high amounts of monounsaturated fat) are excellent quality of oils.

Too much fat, even the good kind, can add excess calories. The U.S. Department of Agriculture (USDA) and the Department of Health and Human Services (HHS) recommend that fat make up no more than 20-35 percent of your daily calories. For example, 20 percent of 1,400 calories equals 280 calories; divided by 9 (the number of calories per gram of fat) is 30 grams of fat.

Polyunsaturated Fats

Poly (or "some", as the name implies) tells us that there will be more than one hydrogen on the carbon chain. Polyunsaturated fats are also liquid at room temperature. Foods high in polyunsaturated fats include vegetable oils such as safflower, corn, sunflower, soy and cottonseed oils. Although these oils are not completely saturated, many times they are partially hydrogenated soybean oil or corn oil.

Laboratory tests have shown that breast tumors appeared more often in animals fed diets high in safflower and corn oil than those fed olive oil. Researchers have also noted higher levels of toxic chemicals such as dichlorodiphenyltrichloroethane (DDT), and polychlorinated biphenyls (PCB) in women with breast cancer. Toxic environmental waste has also been found in fatty tissue. Since the breast is comprised primarily of fatty tissue there is a higher chance of waste being stored there. This means it's not simply the amount or the kind of fat, but what is in it that really counts. That is why fresh or even organic foods may be the best choice.

Omega-3 Fatty Acids

These are a type of polyunsaturated fat that are essential for good health. They are called essential because the body cannot make these fatty acids on its own. Omega-3 must be included in the diet from fatty fish such as salmon, albacore tuna, and mackerel. Another source of omega-3 fatty acid comes from alpha-linoleic acid (ALA), which the body converts into DHA and EPA (docosahexgenoic acid and eicosapentgenoic acid). Alpha –linolenic acid can be found in certain nuts such as walnuts and vegetable oils like canola, soybean, flaxseed, and olive oil.

Include omega-3 in your diet by eating fish at least twice per week and including ground flaxseed in your cereal or salads. You can get flaxseed oil or seeds that have been ground. The seeds must be ground to get the benefit. Whole-seeds can also aid with constipation.

Saturated Fat

Saturated fat is solid at room temperature and mainly in animal products, such as bacon, butter, sour cream, cream cheese, lard, red meat, poultry, and whole cream products. Other main sources contributing to saturated fats that are not from animals include coconut, palm, and other tropical oils.

Trans Fats

Avoid them at all cost. These fats start out as good old unsaturated oils and then are blasted with hydrogen gas to solidify them, creating an acid that raises bad cholesterol and your risk of heart disease. Aim for zero grams on the labels of the foods you bring home. Fortunately and finally, the U.S. Food and Drug Administration (FDA) found partially hydrogenated oils (PHO's) – the primary dietary source of trans fat – unsafe. Manufactures have to eliminate trans fat from their foods.

Moving Our Bodies

Exercise: A commitment to a healthy lifestyle also means getting physically active. Studies have found that people who exercise have a lower risk of developing cancers of the breast and other cancers. Regular activity can help you achieve and maintain a healthy weight, which has also been found to reduce risk of chronic diseases. In preventing cancer initially, the American Institute for Cancer Research reports that women who are physically active have 30 to 40 percent less risk of breast, endometrial, and lung cancers. Regular exercise after breast cancer diagnosis may reduce the risk of death, especially in women with hormone-sensitive tumors, according to the Harvard Nurses' Health Study.

Health Study: Three thousand women with cancer were studied. Those who were physically active by walking three-to-five hours per week at an average pace had the greatest benefit.

The American Cancer Society recommends that we exercise thirty minutes and preferably forty-five to sixty minutes five or more days a week, at a moderate to vigorous pace. Always consult your physician before engaging in any physical activity. Remember to have fun and incorporate a variety of activities like dancing, yoga, playing a sport, Pilates, marathons, or even boot-camp fitness routines. Make it a habit by scheduling it in as a priority. After all, not only does exercise prolong your life, but it reduces daily stress and makes you feel alive and full of stamina.

Moving our bodies and taking the time to do it is an expression of self-love. The new smoking is inactivity. We need to be in harmony and balance with our physical being. Twenty to thirty minutes of exercise should be part of the workday. If it were mandatory we would not have a choice. We would have to do it in order to get our paycheck. Our companies would have stronger, energetic, and healthful employees. We would spend less on medical bills and have fewer sick days. It should be part of our work and healthcare system. Incentives should be given to employees who "work out". A fit staff member is a more productive employee, manager, teacher and they are more effective as executives and professionals.

Any form of moving our bodies' counts: Yoga, Tai chi, Pilates and gentle stretching are beneficial for preventing injuries and for overall health and well-being. Studies on breast cancer have shown that walking as much as five hours a week helps prevent recurring cancer. The most important thing about exercise is that it's an opportunity to have fun and enjoy ourselves with friends and family. So walk, dance, or toss that ball. But do move now. Because while we wait our bodies are slowly but surely breaking down. I ask myself every day, "What kind of 90 year old body do I want to have"? My answer: just like my dad. At age 90, he has never sat for very long and is always walking, biking, stretching, and deep breathing. He's my champion. One of the greatest ways to get up and get moving is the buddy system. In my case, I call it the Kathleen project. Kathleen, my dear, strong, and muscular friend, picks me up at 4:55 a.m. so we can spin, "No Excuses" at 5:15 a.m. I owe her my "work in progress body mode." Her famous words are "give me a month" – somehow this has turned into years. Thanks Kathleen, your body rocks! And so does your inspiration and motivation. Please pick me up for spinning even when we're 90 years old!

A Diet Rich in Wellness

Although there are over 17,500 well- documented diets that exist today, the best diet is one that is rich in phytochemicals and antioxidants – in other words, lots of color. These foods are nature's medicine. Our bodies form free radicals when the body metabolizes oxygen. This is a necessary process to ward off viruses and bacteria. A toxic environment can also promote free radicals. Too many free radicals, and not enough antioxidants can lead to aging and cancer. A combination of phytochemicals or plant chemicals with antioxidants such as (ACE) Vitamin A, vitamin C, and vitamin E should be the fabric of protective and great diet. Phytochemicals can be found in whole grain, beans, fruits, vegetables, nuts, seeds, wine, coffee, tea and dark chocolate.

We are pretty convinced that inflammation is the fire that fuels may diseases including cancer. Inflammation occurs when the immune system is triggered to release chemicals that are damaging, especially when the inflammation occurs for long term. Good nutrition and certain foods can help balance the immune system and insulin levels.

A Mediterranean, Asian, and Indian diet is recommended. All are rich in vegetables, fruits, and vegetable proteins including lentils, peas, beans, and tofu. They also incorporate the use of herbs and spices such as turmeric, mint, thyme, rosemary, and garlic and multi and whole grains like quinoa, bulger, brown rice, and sweet potato.

Choose healthy fats such as olive, canola, flaxseed and Omega-3 oils and butters and eating less animal protein and dairy while opting for more fish and organic meat and eggs. My sister Sandy and I spent some time in Bali and discovered that eating this way gave us enough energy and courage to practice yoga twice a day, meet with the guru and visit three more islands all on the same day. When I remember that trip and the people I met there I am reminded that balance and moderation is the core of wellness.

We can enjoy our favorite foods as long as we incorporate wellness guidelines for our everyday intake. Therefore, limiting alcohol, sweetened drinks, fruit juices, sodas, refined or processed sugars, bleached flours, breads, pastries, muffins, cookies and cakes is a good idea. Something I repeatedly hear in food and nutrition conferences is that help remind me to make better food choices is that sugar kills, but sugar and fat kill faster.

A diet that is focused on wellness and prevention is a diet that is naturally detoxifying and rids the body of carcinogenic substances. It supports the immune system, preventing malnutrition. A powerful diet is one that reduces oxidation, and inflammation to prevent tumor growth and spread. When I am asked about a detox diet my response is always the same. I detox 24/7. Our liver especially is working hard; why not eat a detox diet filled with natural, organic foods that will go to work all day? Eating right is an opportunity to detox 3-5 times a day.

Nutrients that can aid in the body's natural detox process include whole, organic foods, green cruciferous vegetables, probiotics, and adequate filter from beans, whole grains, fruits and nuts. Adding herbs and spices, garlic and onions. Drink green tea and plenty of water.

Whole organic foods – choose foods labeled USDA certified organic. When choosing produce, the USDA has developed a great resource to help you limit your exposure to pesticides. The USDA'S Environmental Working Group (EWG), is a shoppers guide outlining which fruits and vegetables contain the highest amount of pesticides known as their "Dirty Dozen Plus" and also contains a list of which fruits and vegetables contain the least amount of pesticides or not any at all, known as their "Clean Fifteen". Organically grown and raised foods have a positive impact on our health and our environment. Fresh produce can be cleaned by mixing a solution of 16 oz.

water and 2 table spoons of vinegar for 2-3 minutes and then rinse and brush.

Functional Food

It is a very exciting time for the science of nutrition. For years we have focused on what foods we should avoid. But today, research is revealing a lot more about the benefits of certain foods that have a potentially positive effect on health beyond basic nutrition. These are called functional foods. These foods contain phytochemicals – and "phyto" means plant. These plant substances fight for our health. They are also called super foods.

Just as the public developed an interest a hundred years ago about the discovery of vitamins, today we are seeing great enthusiasm as scientist explore the "functional" benefits of phytonutrients. They provoke health by slowing the aging process and reducing the risk for chronic diseases. They are bioactive substances that plants produce naturally to protect themselves against viruses and bacteria. There are thousands of phytonutrients, providing aroma and flavor to our foods. At least two thousand are responsible for plant pigments that make the food on our plates burst with color.

One orange may have more than 150 different phytonutrients. Carotenoids give oranges their bright color. Flavonoids give blueberries their blue tint. Both act as antioxidants and may neutralize free radicals. Quercetin, found in tea, onions, and other vegetables may reduce the growth and spread of cancer cells. Plant-based foods contain a variety of these protective substances, especially fruits and vegetables. Phytonutrients are grouped according to their characteristics and possible protective function (see List 1, Examples of Functional Components for functional nutrition phytonutrient list), Other foods that may lower cancer risk include catechins in white, oolong, green, or black tea, which on the oxygen-radical absorbency capacity (ORAC) score ranked as high or higher in antioxidant potential than many fruits and vegetables.

Researchers at the University of Rochester, New York Medical Center have found that EGCG, another antioxidant component in green tea, has an affinity for a common protein in cancer cell, which may prevent the cascade of events that triggers cancer. The way EGCG may stop the cancer process before it starts is by interfering with some of the processes involved in cell replication, which kill tumor cell. My coauthor Cindy and I have tea together all the time. These foods mentioned above along with many other ones in research today are most likely to have cancer-fighting potential.

It is important not to obsess about any one specific food. There is no single food that can prevent cancer. There are dietary strategies, however that can help make a difference.

Consuming a broad range of healthful foods and living a new, improved lifestyle is smart. A smart lifestyle includes not smoking. Talking to trained professionals about the best option to quit is crucial. Also avoid exposure to sun on your skin, but do get enough vitamin D, "the sunshine vitamin", Research tell us to avoid sun exposure between 10:00 A.M. and 2:00 P.M., Researchers also recommend protecting your skin with clothing or sunscreen.

Vitamin D is absorbed within just a few minutes of sun, several days, or a week. Consume fortified milk or fatty fish. If you do not get some sun or consume milk or fatty fish then consider taking a multivitamin with vitamin D or any other vitamin D supplement. There is mounting evidence that vitamin D may protect against several types of cancers including breast cancer.

Super Survivor Food

Broccoli: My favorite! I chop it up and put it in everything including beans, quinoa, and even hummus spread. Along with kale, brussel sprouts, cauliflower and cabbage, broccoli has been extensively studied by scientists. The general consensus is that the chemicals in the cruciferous family can ward off and protect against cancer. Broccoli contains a much-researched chemical called glucosinolates, which breaks into indoles and isothiocyanates. It appears to be protecting against hormone–related cancers like breast cancer. The chemical indoles interrupt the replication of cancer cells. That is why broccoli has become one of my favorite medicinal foods. I call it my daily dose.

Paul Talalay, M.D., professor of pharmacology and molecular science at Johns Hopkins University in Baltimore was one of the scientists who discovered the potent cancer-fighting isothiocyanate sulforaphane in broccoli (try saying that five times fast!). He also found that tender broccoli sprouts are a superrich source of sulforaphane. According to Dr. Talalay, broccoli and other cruciferous vegetables such as cabbage, kale, cauliflower, and brussel sprouts have anticancer substances: When plant cells are broken down during chewing, glucosinolates are released and converted to another protective substance called isothiocyantes. These chemicals induce enzymes that help detoxification and boost antioxidants, says Dr. Talalay. Other colorful vegetables with protective properties include tomatoes, squash, carrots, and dark leafy greens.

Probiotics - Friendly Bacteria: The health of our gut is crucial in the healing and prevention of diseases; the colon holds unfriendly bacteria and free radicals. Therefore, we must create a good environment in the gut for good health. Eating more fiber, drinking plenty of water and getting a probiotic supplement will make for a happy gastrointestinal tract. Always consult with your physician or dietician before staring any supplement.

Berries: I am wild about berries! I promote them daily for their wide range of phytochemicals, high fiber, and vitamin C. They are sweet, juicy, and a bit tart at times which makes them perfect to pair with a variety of foods such as vanilla yogurt, salads and as relish on chicken and fish dishes. The variety is abundant. You can choose from wild blueberries, which have about 26 antioxidants to salmonberries, which are part of the rose family. They are pink, salmon colored, but turned red as they ripen. They are not easy to find but exquisite. The darker berries like blackberries and blueberries are literally under the microscope. Scientists are telling us that the phytochemicals and antioxidants may be potential cancer fighters. I buy a variety of fresh berries and freeze them so I can enjoy them all year round. I make warm berry desserts natural jams, relish, and even salad dressings with berries.

Seeds are the future. They take our food supply to the next generation and contain a concentration of nutrients and oils that are full of flavor, texture and nutritional benefits. I sprinkle, stir, grind, and crunch on seeds like chia, flax, hemp, pumpkin, sesame, sunflower, and watermelon.

Seeds are rich with minerals and healthful fats such as polyunsaturated fatty acids. I grew up watering my chia pet and now I eat them because they are packed with protein, omega–3 fatty acids, fiber, and minerals such as iron, calcium, magnesium, and manganese. Chia makes an excellent nonfat thickener for soups and sauces. The gelatinous paste is a type of soluble fiber that is important in heart health.

Flax seeds are bursting with powerful antioxidants, omega-3 fatty acids, protein and vitamin B, zinc, magnesium and manganese. It's important to grind the flaxseed; otherwise it passes through the digestive tract intact. I sprinkle ground golden flaxseed on my oatmeal, berry smoothies, salads, soups, beans, and quinoa berry muffins.

Hemp seeds are getting lots of attention for its high protein and excellent omega-3 fatty acid and mineral content I sprinkle them over yogurt, cereal and savory dishes like stir–fry and soups. Toasting them a bit before you eat or cook with them makes them tastier.

Herbs and the Spice of Life

Spices are the easiest way to become creative in the kitchen; they help me cut back on fat for taste. The ancient healers have used them all across the world. They have exchanged them as medicines in the form of tinctures, teas, syrups, oils and extracts. Scientists today have found they may have phytochemicals that are antioxidant, anti-inflammatory and protect against bacteria and viruses.

Buy fresh rosemary, thyme, oregano, basil, mint and ginger, which are super, fragrant and aromatic when you cook them. Turmeric and curry, native to the orient, have been cultivated for at least 5,000 years in India. They are also found in the Caribbean and are the most powerful natural anti-inflammatories identified by scientists at the moment. Studies are emerging with news about turmeric's main compound, curcumin. This compound has been found to be helpful in playing a role against many diseases including Alzheimer's. It has been shown that curcumin may inhibit the growth of certain cancers. It's the anti-inflammatory and antioxidant spice. Its warm, golden color livens every stew, soup, chili, casserole and salad in my kitchen. At the top of the list for inhibiting the most cancers, including breast cancer, are garlic, leeks, scallions, and ginger root – all powerful anti-inflammatories and antioxidants.

Ginger tea eases nausea from chemotherapy and the side effects of radiation. I get creative and combine olive oil, turmeric, black pepper, garlic, leeks, wild blue berries, scallions, ginger, and balsamic vinegar for a cancer-fighting dressing I use on my salads and vegetable dishes. It was a favorite among my colleagues when I worked at a hospital. You can add plain yogurt and turn it into a super dip.

Dark Chocolate, Red Wine, Coffee and Self Love

Dark Chocolate

I've always had a passion for dark chocolate; however my true love affair began in a small island called Sao Tome and Principe, Africa's second-smallest country. I was there on a health mission with my husband when I gained a deep appreciation for cocoa beans. I learned that chocolate means bitter water and that the Aztecs made a bitter drink from cocoa beans and spices. The Mayans believed the bitter drink would heal their hearts, minds and bodies. Now scientific research has revealed a type of anti-oxidant and phytochemical called catechins and flavonoids. These compounds are getting kudos for heart health. The Mayans may have been on to something sweet, while sipping their bitter cocoa drink. I've noticed that a piece of dark chocolate a day makes me happy, wholesome, and very satisfied.

Red Wine

For many of us wine lovers, there is not much convincing to be done here. Wine is a decadent and honorable socialite. It's also noteworthy for the great scientific evidence linking the phytochemical, resveratrol to a multitude of health benefits especially for decreasing risk of coronary disease and stroke. The powerful resveratrol has demonstrated to have antioxidant, anti-clotting, anti-inflammatory, and anti-cancer properties.

Alcohol

This is another subject that needs to be addressed because research is now saying that women who consume even a few drinks per week have an increased risk for breast cancer. The reason is that alcohol may raise estrogen levels, which increases the risk of breast cancer. According to the Nurses' Health Study, the increased risk for breast cancer link with alcohol occurs mostly in women who don't get adequate amounts of the B vitamin and folic acid. Limit alcohol drinks to one per day. However, women who have had breast cancer are at high risk should avoid alcohol altogether. Because there is evidence that alcohol may protect against heart disease, ask your physician if drinking in moderation may benefit or increase risk, based on your genetic predisposition.

Coffee

The aroma is captivating, alluring and as many of us know, addicting. With good varieties of coffee beans it's easy to fall and stay in love. Coffee beans have over 1,000 active compounds, phyto chemicals and a high anti-oxidant profile. The health benefits range from improved mental, and physical performance to cancer fighting properties. One analysis of eight studies on endometrial cancer risk and coffee involving 300,000 women, found a decrease of seven percent risk in developing endometrial cancer. Another good reason to enjoy a cup of Jo.

H2O

Humans are made up of mostly water. The average person carries 10 to 12 gallons of it. It is essential in digestion and excretion. It lubricates our joints and is a major component of body fluids. It is our natural, calorie free, cleansing and purifying drink. The most beautiful skin and balanced body's carry it in abundance. Dehydration causes headaches, increased appetite, constipation, irritability, and lethargy. We cannot live without and would die in its absence in a few days. With the incredible burden we put on our kidneys, from toxins and pollutants from our environment it is a shame that for most people it's a struggle to get the recommended 8-8oz glasses per day. I have found that recommending drinking a couple of glasses of water in the afternoon helps as a pick-me up, much like when you water a dying plant and it quickly comes back to life.

Although calorie-free, somehow it energizes me. It also helps to curb my appetite during those hungry hours from 3 p.m. to 6 p.m. until dinner is ready. I call these the witches hours because if were not careful we can eat right through the pantry. A combination of accumulated stress from the day, appetite, and running around to wrap up our daily routine can create cause for over eating, even though we have probably consumed a pristine diet all day. I found eating a substantial, nutrient-dense snack and hydrating with water was the answer. During these hours it is a good idea to have a healthy snack on hand and pair it up with a nice tall glass of infused H2o. I love natural infusions of lemon or berries in my water but there is nothing like pure, crystal-clear, cleansing H2o.

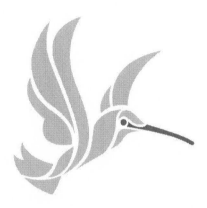

Wellness Meal Plan

These meal plans were designed using a variety of foods rich in phytochemical, anti-oxidants, omega-3 fatty acids and rich in vitamins and minerals. To promote clean eating by choose a variety of super and functional foods that are farm fresh, organic, non-GMO and minimally or non-processed foods. Always check the first ingredient in your foods, that's what you are eating most of.

Garlic, leeks, onions, shallots, herbs, turmeric, curry, omega rich oils, and low-fat dairy products, are foods that you should use often. Be sure to wash all fruits, vegetables and salads thoroughly and remove outer leaves to reduce exposure to pesticides.

DAY 1
Breakfast
1 cup oatmeal

¾ cup wild blueberries

12 almonds, slivered

8 oz. 0-1% fat milk, Almond or cashew milk

1 cup green tea

Lunch

2 slices light rye bread

2 oz. turkey breast nitrite free

1 oz. low-fat Swiss cheese

1 teaspoon olive oil mayo sprinkle turmeric makes

1 teaspoon mustard

½ cup baby carrots

2 tablespoons nonfat Greek yogurt dressing for carrots

2 kiwis

Snack

1 cup nonfat light fruit yogurt

12 cherries, sweet or fresh

1 tablespoons flaxseed

Dinner

1 cup brown wild rice

1 cup zucchini plus 5 tablespoons chopped /cooked onions

1 cup summer squash

4-6 oz. wild Alaskan salmon grilled, baked, broiled, or pan –fried

1 teaspoon coconut oil for cooking salmon

DAY 2

Breakfast

1 protein bar

½ cup pomegranate juice

1 cup low-fat light vanilla yogurt

Lunch

2 eight –inch whole corn tortillas

7 oz. grilled chicken cut into strips

½ cup fresh or already prepared salsa (chopped tomato, scallions, cilantro in a tomato sauce, sprinkle turmeric) over grilled chicken.

1 cup shredded kale or spinach in tortillas

1 cup mixed fresh berries-strawberries, blackberries, or raspberries add balsamic vinegar a dash of agave and freeze.

Snack

7 walnuts

1 cup white tea with fresh ginger

Dinner

8 oz. sautéed shrimp in marinara sauce

Marinara sauce, use lots of chopped up heirloom tomatoes

Leeks /shallots

3 cloves garlic

2 teaspoons olive oil

1 cup fresh tomatoes

1 cup ready-made tomato pasta sauce, low- fat

2 cups linguini or gluten free pasta

2 tablespoons grated parmesan cheese

1 cup broccoli, steamed

DAY 3

Breakfast

Almond smoothie

1 cup milk, vanilla almond milk

1 ¼ cup strawberries to mix in blender. May use variation of frozen or fresh fruit. Peaches are an excellent stone fruit.

Lunch

1 serving of seed crackers

3 oz. canned tuna

1 tablespoon reduced-fat mayonnaise to mix with tuna, sprinkle turmeric

Chop scallions, leeks and black pepper

2 sliced plum tomatoes, baby spinach leaves, chopped onions

½ cup frozen yogurt
Snack
1 green apple cut into slices, powdered with cinnamon
1 tsp of almond butter
Dinner
5 oz. veggie burger
¼ cup mushrooms, ¼ cup onions, ¼ cup red bell peppers,
sautéed with 1 teaspoon of olive oil and dried spices of choice.
1 cup brown rice with veggies
½ cup black beans
7 spears fresh asparagus
½ cup frozen mango

DAY 4
Breakfast
1 cup high –fiber cereal
1 small banana
8 oz. of 1% milk almond, cashew milk.
Lunch
Mini pizza
1 whole grain pita bread
½ cup tomato sauce
½ cup chopped tomatoes
3 oz. light mozzarella cheese
½ cup mixed veggies on top lots of chopped broccoli
1 slice apricot sprinkled with low-fat granola and a tablespoon of
vanilla yogurt
Snack
Fresh large pear and a piece of dark chocolate
Dinner
8 oz. flounder, baked
1 teaspoon olive oil
Minced fresh garlic, scallions, leeks

1 large sweet potato

1 cup green beans

1 baked apple with low-fat vanilla frozen yogurt

Sautéed the olive oil with the fresh garlic and pour over the fish.

DAY 5

Breakfast

3 egg whites (cooked to your choice)

¼ cup fresh mushrooms, sliced

¼ cup chopped onions

¼ cup diced tomato

¼ cup diced red, green, or yellow bell peppers

1 tablespoon olive oil to sautéed the vegetables to mix with the egg whites

1 oz. low-fat cheese

4 oz. orange juice

2 slices whole –grain toast

Lunch

1 sweet potato with chives

4 oz. organic chicken strips

1 spinach salad

½ cup grape tomatoes

1 cup watermelon

Snack

1 cup low-fat blueberry yogurt or ½ cup fresh blueberries

Dinner

5 oz. eggplant parmesan cheese with cooked garlic spinach

7 asparagus spears

½ cup banana

¼ cup frozen grapes

¼ cup strawberries

½ cup low-fat vanilla yogurt

DAY 6

Breakfast

Pumpernickel bagel

½ teaspoon cashew butter

4 oz. blueberry juice

8 oz. low –fat milk or yogurt

Lunch

4 oz. roasted chicken

1 cup of quinoa

Add all ingredients below to quinoa

2 teaspoon of slithered almonds

2 teaspoon of golden raisins

1 cup of mixed veggies

1 teaspoon of turmeric with ½ teaspoon black pepper

garlic, pearl, onions, shallots, leeks.

Snack

¼ cup high –fiber cereal

½ cup low-fat vanilla yogurt

1 teaspoon honey, drizzled over cereal and yogurt

Dinner

6 oz. baked grouper

1 cup steamed broccoli with garlic and herbs

1 sweet potato

Romaine lettuce, green /red/yellow bell peppers chopped, cucumbers, tomatoes, onions, light vinaigrette dressing

1 cup of ginger tea

DAY 7

Breakfast

1 cup oatmeal

1 cup chopped fresh blackberries

1 teaspoon cinnamon

4 oz. pomegranate juice

Lunch

Bean vegetable soup (buy a combination of beans and mix)

Add onions, garlic, fresh herbs and seasonings to beans

Whole grain /pumpkin seed crackers

1 cup cherries

Snacks

1 protein bar

1 cup of jasmine green tea

Dinner

2 cups quinoa pasta

1 tablespoon olive oil.

4 oz. shrimp lightly pan-fried with black pepper and salt.

2 tablespoon parmesan cheese

1 cup spinach leaves with ½ cup strawberries in a raspberry vinaigrette sauce, sprinkle walnuts

DAY 8

Breakfast

1 flat whole grain bread

1 tablespoon almond butter

1 egg. Sunny side up

2 strips turkey, thin sliced and pan-fried with olive oil spray

4 oz. blueberry juice

Lunch

4 oz. smoked salmon with tomato and onion on a bagel

1 teaspoon low-fat cream cheese

2 cups green lettuce mixed with grated carrots, beets, cucumbers

Snacks

1 protein bar/ dipped in 1 tablespoon of honey peanut butter

1 cup of tea

Dinner

1 cup vegetable or bean soup with a variety of mixed veggies chopped in.

1 whole-wheat grain roll or seed crackers

3oz. grilled chicken with diced mango and onions on top, on a bed of thinly sliced avocado

1 piece of dark chocolate

. . .

DAY 9

Breakfast

1 cup veggie omelet, spinach, broccoli, onions, shallots, leeks

1 cup almond cashew milk

½ cup raspberries

Lunch

1 cup tuna salad

2 slices whole grain /whole oat bread

1 teaspoon reduced-fat mayonnaise add turmeric

2 cups leafy greens like kale or broccoli

1 tablespoon olive oil with balsamic vinegar

1 cup green tea

Snack

1 protein bar

1cup of mango or papaya green tea

Dinner

1 cup lean beef or turkey chili, beans in a bowl with lettuce, tomato, onions, shredded low fat, cheddar cheese

1 cup steamed mixed vegetables

DAY 10

Breakfast

6 oz. grape juice

1 cup fresh strawberries

8 oz. low-fat almond cashew milk

1 tsp. vanilla

Oat muffins mix 1 cup oats and ¾ coconut floor, 1 ½ baking soda,
½ cup chopped walnuts
Bake 350° - 20-30 min, or until firm.

Lunch

8 oz. grilled Mahi Mahi

2 slices of whole –grain bread or roll

1 teaspoon tartar sauce

2 stalks of bok choy

1 cup tomato wedges and sliced onions

1 tablespoon salad dressing made with olive oil and balsamic
vinegar

Snack

3 cups air-popped popcorn sprinkled with garlic powder and herbs.

Dinner

3 oz. broiled pork tenderloin

1 cup wild rice with mixed veggies

1 cup steamed broccoli

½ cup frozen fruit dessert

1 cup green tea

DAY 11

Breakfast

8 oz. green drink, kale spinach, green apple, ginger

1 cup cooked oatmeal with 2 tablespoons raisins

1 cup fresh blueberries

1 cup soy or low –fat milk

Lunch

8 oz. Baked halibut

1 cup wild rice with crushed walnuts, spice it up with tarragon and turmeric

1 cup mixed vegetables.

Snack

1 protein bar

Dinner

Broccoli, hemp soup, blended with, 1 large carrot, onion,

1 cup ginger or chicken,

1 tablespoon leeks, broth,

3 tablespoon hemp seeds

1 piece dark chocolate

DAY 12

Breakfast

2 Oat Pancakes, with 1 large sliced baked apple with cinnamon

¼ cup real fruit compote

6 oz. fruit smoothie , made in blender with ½ cup blueberries , 6 oz. vanilla soy milk , and ice

1tsp Chia Seeds

Lunch

1 chicken sandwich with 2 whole grain wrap, lettuce, tomato, onions, 1 tablespoon low-fat mayonnaise add turmeric

1 piece dark chocolate

Snack

½ cup Greek yogurt with Blackberries, blueberries and Slithers of Almonds

Dinner

1 cup quinoa pasta primavera

½ cup marinara sauce with chopped spinach and 3 oz. shrimp or scallops

1 cup mixed veggies in sauce

½ cup frozen grapes

1 cup diced strawberries, orange, kiwi or mangoes

More Recipes

Mediterranean Leafy Salmon

(1-2 Servings)

Ingredients:
10 cups mixed organic leafy greens
8 oz. salmon
¾ cup crumbled feta cheese (if desired)
1 small sliced and cooked red bell pepper
4 sliced black olives
Salt and pepper to taste
2 tablespoons raspberry vinaigrette –sprinkle with 2 tablespoons of sliced almonds, if desired
Preparation:
Grill or bake salmon
Toss all ingredients and enjoy in a chilled bowl. Garnish with parsley leaf

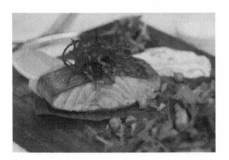

Mediterranean Leafy Salmon
Mediterranean leafy salmon is not only exquisite in taste, but it

also looks beautiful. It's like having a fruit festival on a plate. The combination of salmon and red bell peppers with black olives is very special. Salmon is rich in Omega -3 fatty acids, making it a heart healthy choice. The leafy greens and crumbled feta cheese makes this recipe appropriate for mid –day or evening. Enjoy especially under candlelight.

Pumpkin Soup: (Servings, 1 Cup each)

Ingredients

1 large Vidalia onion

2 garlic cloves

2 cup pumpkin, canned or fresh

6 cups chicken broth and a pinch of cumin powder and curry ½ teaspoon of allspice.

Pinch of salt

1 cup coconut milk or low-fat plain yogurt

Chopped leeks

PREPARATION:

Boil all ingredients except milk in a pot.

Simmer for 20 minutes and let cool.

Puree soup in a blender and return to pot.

Add skim or low-fat milk and stir.

Place a dapple of low-fat plain yogurt in the middle of the soup, in each bowl, if desired.

Garnish with leeks.

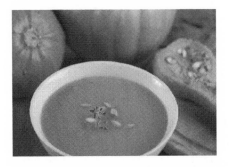

Nutrition Analysis:

Per Serving: 145 calories, 2 gm fat, 6 gm protein, 2 gm carbohydrates, 3 mg cholesterol

Pumpkin Soup is rich in beta-carotene. Research suggests that its antioxidant properties may protect against some cancers. Beta-carotene functions in immunity, vision, taste/smell, wound healing, and skin integrity.

It is also found in carrots, sweet potatoes, apricots, cantaloupe, pink grapefruit, and other orange winter squash. This delicious soup also contains calcium, which is needed for bone and tooth structure, bone absorption, and blood clotting. This soup is easy to prepare, looks great, and tastes amazing. Enjoy!

Broccolini A La Houdini: (2 Servings, 1 cup each)

Ingredients:

4 oz. multigrain or quinoa pasta

2 cups fresh broccoli

4 medium carrots

2 cups vegetable broth

4 garlic cloves

1 small onion

1 tablespoon of olive oil

2 tablespoons grated Fresh Parmesan cheese

Preparation:

Boil pasta as directed on package.

Put broccoli, carrots, vegetable broth, garlic, onion, and olive oil in blender; chop and mix all together. Heat in saucepan and pour over pasta. Sprinkle with parmesan cheese. Garnish with basil leaf.

Nutrition Analysis:

Per Serving: 350 calories, 7 gm fat, 12 gm protein, 38 gm carbohydrates, 2 mg cholesterol

Broccoli a la Houdini

Broccoli a la Houdini is an amazing recipe for those who do not put broccoli at the top of their favorite food list. The vegetable disappears when you blend it. However, the benefits remain.

Broccoli is known as one of the healthiest foods used by mankind. Experts agree that cruciferous vegetables contain cancer-fighting components. Cruciferous vegetables also include bok choy, brussel sprouts, cabbage, cauliflower, and more. Enjoy this recipe as you benefit from the increase of veggies in your diet.

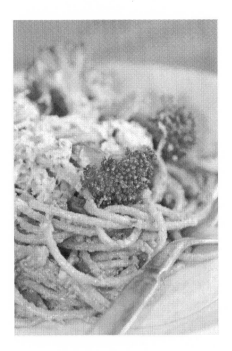

Tangy Three –Bean Salad: (2-3 Servings)

Ingredients:

½ cup small white beans
½ cup red Kidney beans
½ cup garbanzo beans
¾ cup sliced green onions
¾ cup sliced black olives
3 garlic cloves, chopped
3 tablespoons of feta cheese, sprinkled
3 tablespoons olive oil
3 tablespoons cilantro chopped
½ teaspoon of hot sauce if desired, with ½ teaspoon of salt
1 ½ cups Romaine lettuce

Preparation:

Cook beans (can also use canned). Sauté green onions, garlic, olive oil, and salt. Mix the beans into the pan with the sauté and add cilantro and hot sauce to taste. Garnish with lemon slices and parsley leaf.

Nutrition Analysis:

Per Serving: 240 calories, 3 gm fat, 21 g, protein, 30 gm carbohydrates, 3mg cholesterol

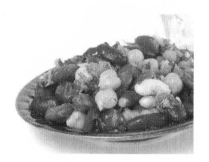

TANGY THREE –BEAN SALAD

Dried beans or legumes are the best plant source of protein that nature provides. Beans are also an excellent source of soluble fiber, which has been shown to aid in lowering cholesterol and controlling blood sugar. Insoluble fiber is also present, which increases bulk and alleviates some digestive problems. Beans are also known for being a good source of iron. This recipe is an ideal alternative to meat. Serve with a little rice to make it a complete protein and enjoy.

Cannon Ball Smoothie: (2-3 8-oz SERVINGS)

Ingredients:

½ cup frozen or fresh blueberries (wild blueberries have 26 antioxidants)

½ cup frozen or fresh strawberries

1/2 cup greek vanilla yogurt

1/2 cup pomegranate juice

1 tablespoon flaxseed or chia seeds
1 scoop protein powder, if desired
Preparation:
Mix all ingredients in a blender and serve chilled.

Nutrition Analysis:

Per Serving: 220 calories, 1 gm fat, 7 gm protein (24 gm with protein powder), 45 gm carbohydrates,

0 mg cholesterol

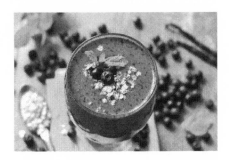

The Cannon Ball Smoothie can be made with just about any berry you like. Berries are full of vitamin C, potassium, fiber, and flavonoids, which research shows may bolster cellular antioxidant defenses. This recipe also contains calcium for strong bones and teeth, and flaxseed, a source of omega 3 fatty acids, and may contribute to maintaining of heart health research has shown.

An excellent way to start your day or even enjoy as a midday snack.

Wicked Food

The wicked, keep way low or way-out

The foods below should not be part of our regular everyday diet. Consuming these foods in excess may cause inflammation which science tells us play a key role in the development of diseases. There are creative ways of making many of these foods using fresh fruit and alternative natural sweeteners. Always avoid:

GMO
    Processed
    Artificial
    Trans Fats
    Hydrogenated oils
    Fried
    Chargrilled
    Hormones
    Refined Sugar
    Excess white flour, Rice, Pasta, Potato
    Candy
    Cookies,
    Cupcakes
    Cakes
    Pies
    Pastries
    Jelly, Jams, Syrup
    Sodas
    Juices
    Sugar drinks
    Excess Alcohol
    Vegetable oils, corn soybean, sunflower
    Eggs from poor caged chickens
    Excess animal protein

Remember, excess sugar kills. Excess sugar and fat--kill faster.

Excess calories no matter where they come from get stored as fat and cause excess weight.

Be mindful of the way foods make you feel. Go for super foods, leave the wicked out. Use aromatic oils as scents to soothe emotions instead of going for the sugar.

The Healthy Pantry

Here is a quick grocery list, to ensure you always have plenty of healthy options

STARCHES	FRUITS
Quinoa	Wild Blueberries
Sweet potato	Raspberries
Seed crackers	Pomegranate Juice
Oats	Strawberries
Bulgur	Any stone-bearing fruit like apricots
Multi grain bread	Cherries
Flat Bread and pita	black berries
	organic apples

VEGGIES	FATS
Broccoli	Fish Oils/Omega 3
Kale	Flaxseed oil
Spinach	Linseed oil
Cauliflower	Olive Oil
Squash	Fatty Acid
Pumpkin	Coconut oil virgin
Peppers all colors	
Cucumbers	
Tomatoes	
Eggplant	

SPICES

Basil
Chives
Cilantro
Garlic
Ginger
Mint
Pepper
Rosemary
Thyme
Turmeric
Vanilla

DAIRY

Omega 3 grass fed
Non-GMO
Organic dairy eggs

PROTEIN

Fish
Shellfish
Tuna
Sardines
Cage Free eggs
Lentil and colors beans
Tofu and tempeh
Greek Yogurt

SEEDS and NUTS

Hemp
Chia
Flax
Pumpkin
Almonds
Walnuts
Cashews

SUGARS

Agave Nectar
Stevia
Acacia Honey

EXTRA PLEASURE

Green Tea
Dark chocolate
Your favorite protein bars

Be mindful of your mealtime. It is a sacred time of nourishment. Over eating happens when we are not connected to our core. Take a deep breath and be thankful before your meals. Eating is a ritual, a pleasure that if respected will in turn provide our bodies with all the nourishment we need even in our soul and spirit. I invite you to practice the art of mindful eating and become more aware of your behavior with food; know when your body has reached the point of satisfaction and do not eat beyond that point. We are constantly making food choices. If you eat three meals a day, you have 90 opportunities a month to consciously make better choices to improve our nutrition.

Going through a Cancer Diagnosis

All aspects of wellbeing are associated with proper nutrition. It is important to note, if you are already faced with a cancer diagnosis, seek individual medical nutrition therapy by a registered dietitian/nutritionist. A nutritionist will properly assess your individual needs and tailor a meal plan for you to follow. Nutritionists have special training to help you find the path to properly nourish yourself from at the cellular level.

When I found my mother had been diagnosed with breast cancer, it turned my world upside down. I lost my appetite for a few days, and for months. A cancer diagnosis can have this effect on the people going through it, and on those who love and care for them. Make an effort to make good nutrition a priority at this time. It is essential to helping you feel better and stronger.

I learned from my mother's experience that proper nutrition helps you handle the side effects of cancer treatment. Eating right also reduces your chances of infection and assists with your recovery from treatment or surgery. Keep foods fresh and be sure to practice safe food handling because your immune response may not be as optimal. When white blood cells are low the body has a harder time fighting infection or harmful bacteria.

During treatment with chemotherapy and radiation therapy, you may have friends and family who offer all kinds of advice on complementary or alternative therapies, vitamins, minerals, herbal products, and have miracle potions. They have good intentions and it is reassuring to know that your loved ones are taking a proactive role in your care. However, be cautious because while some of these products may be safe and harmless and others are not. They may interfere

with the effects of radiation of chemotherapy. Some may even interfere with recovery from surgery and others may have harmful side
effects. Be sure to consult your physician, your dietitian or both about
any alternative or complementary therapies.

I am grateful to share that my dear mom, Maribella is doing
awesome. We celebrate her life by taking her on fun adventures that
include riding camels. During her cancer treatment, she joked "If I
survive this one, I'll ride a camel through the desert." So, my sister
Sandy and I took her on an adventure through the deserts of Egypt
and a camel she rode.

References

1. A very warm and special thank you to Claudia Miro my
friend and professional Hispanic translator and language
specialist from Rapid Pro, for her expertise in reviewing
and editing my chapter.

2. Psychology Today - "6 Lessons We Can Learn From
Eastern Chinese Medicine." https://www.psychologytoday.
com/blog/the-doctor-is-listening/201301/6-lessons-we-can-
learn-eastern-chinese-medicine

3. Academy of Nutrition and Dietetics - Eat Right:
http://www.eatright.org/

4. American Cancer Society: http://www.cancer.org/

5. American Diabetes Association®: http://www.
diabetes.org/

6. American Heart Association: http://www.
heart.org/HEARTORG/

7. American Institute for Cancer Research (AICR) – "Protein
vs Carbohydrates: A Weight Loss Choice?" http://
preventcancer.aicr.org/site/News2?page=NewsArticle&id=
7462&news_iv_ctrl=0&abbr=pub_

8. Hopkins Medicine.org: "Cancer Protection Compound

Abundant in Broccoli Sprouts." http://www.
hopkinsmedicine.org/press/1997/SEPT/970903.HTM

9. Web MD.com: "Cancer-Fighting Foods: Diet to Help
   Prevent Cancer." http://www.webmd.com/diet/eating-
   good-health

10. Cancer.gov: "Eating Hints: Before, During, and After
    Cancer Treatment." http://www.cancer.gov/publications/
    patient-education/eatinghints.pdf

11. Chicago Tribune: "Environmental Nutrition: Celebrate
    Cruciferous Vegetables." http://www.chicagotribune.com/
    lifestyles/food/sns-201508311800--tms--foodstylts--v-
    f20150831-20150831-story.html

12. USDA.gov: "Food and Nutrition." http://www.usda.gov/
    wps/portal/usda/usdahome?navid=food-nutrition

13. "Food Circles: Envisioning How Eating a Variety of Foods
    Over Time Will Benefit Health." *The Journal of Integrative
    Medicine & Therapy* 1.1 (2014). Print

14. Hummingwell.com: "Tips." http://www.
    hummingwell.com/tips/

15. Food Insight.org: "IFIC Foundation - Your Nutrition and
    Food Safety Resource." http://www.foodinsight.org/

16. India Diets.com: "Health, Nutrition, Fitness, Weight Loss."
    http://www.indiadiets.com/

17. http://www.mindful.org

18. EPA.gov: "Organic Farming | Agriculture | US EPA."

19. http://www.epa.gov/agriculture/torg.html

20. Que Flaca, Fuerte y Feliz http://www.queflaca.com @que
    flaca

21. Sabrina Hernandez (@hummingwell) | Twitter.

22. Sabrina Hernandez, RD, LD/N, CDE Dietitian /
    Nutritionist:

23. http://www.hummingwell.com/sabrina-hernandez-cano/

24. PBS.org: "The Dirty Dozen and Clean 15 of Produce | Need
    to Know | PBS."

25. http://www.pbs.org/wnet/need-to-know/health/the-dirty-dozen-and-clean-15-of-produce/616/
26. U.S. News & World Report: "Traditional Asian Diet -- What You Need to Know."
27. http://health.usnews.com/best-diet/traditional-asian-diet
28. FDA.gov: "Trans Fat - Food and Drug Administration." http://www.fda.gov/NewsEvents/Newsroom/PressAnnouncements/ucm451237.htm
29. US Environmental Protection Agency. http://www.epa.gov
30. "USDA Nutrition Research Focuses on Cancer Killing Compounds." *Rodale's All-new Encyclopedia of Organic Gardening.* 1997. Print.
31. Duyff, Roberta Larson. *American Dietetic Association Complete Food and Nutrition Guide.* Hoboken, NJ: John Wiley & Sons, 2006. Print.
32. Elk, Ronit, and Monica Morrow. *Breast Cancer for Dummies.* Hoboken, NJ: Wiley Pub., 2003. Print.
33. Friedman, Rodney M., and Sheldon Margen. *Wellness Foods A-Z an Indispensable Guide for Health-conscious Food Lovers.* New York: Rebus, 2002. Print.
34. Koch, Maryjo. *Seed Leaf Flower Fruit.* San Francisco: Collins San Francisco, 1995. Print.
35. McKay, Judith, and Tamera Schacher. *The Chemotherapy Survival Guide: Everything You Need to Know to Get through Treatment.* Oakland, CA: New Harbinger Publications, 2009. Print.
36. Papale-Hammontree, Cindy, and Sabrina Hernandez. *The Empty Cup Runneth Over: Answers about Breast Cancer from the Experts.* Pittsburgh, PA: Dorrance Pub., 2008. Print.
37. Peto, Richard. "The Causes of Cancer: Quantitative Estimates of Avoidable Risks of Cancer in the United States Today." *The Use of Human Cells for the Evaluation of Risk from Physical and Chemical Agents* (1983): 587-93. Print.
38. Quillin, Patrick, and Noreen Quillin. *Beating Cancer with*

Nutrition: Combining the Best of Science and Nature for Healing in the 21st Century: Simple, Safe, and Effective Natural Methods to Improve Outcome for Cancer Patients. Tulsa, OK: Nutrition Times, 2001. Print.

39. Rosenthal, Joshua. *Integrative Nutrition: Feed Your Hunger for Health and Happiness*. New York, NY: Integrative Nutrition Pub., 2008. Print.

40. Sawyer, Allie Fair., and Norma Suzette. Jones. *Journey: A Breast Cancer Survival Guide*. Alexander, NC: WorldComm, 1992. Print.

41. Servan-Schreiber, David. *Anti Cancer: A New Way of Life*. Melbourne, Australia: Scribe, 2008. Print.

42. Varona, Verne. *Nature's Cancer-fighting Foods: Prevent and Reverse the Most Common Forms of Cancer Using the Proven Power of Great Food and Easy Recipes*. Paramus, NJ: Reward, 2001. Print.

~

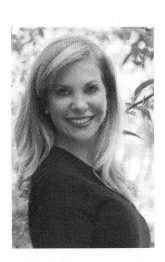

Sabrina Hernandez-Cano, a Registered & licensed Dietitian, Nutrition Counselor, and Certified Diabetes Educator, graduated from Florida International University with a degree in Dietetics & Nutrition. Celebrating

25 years as member of the Academy of Nutrition and Dietetics, she has served as President of the Miami Dietetic Association and voted The Greater Miami Dietitian Award.

Sabrina received the Miami Herald Silver Knight Award for founding , 'Heart lights", a movement that helped feed and shelter the homeless and hungry in Hialeah, her hometown where she was born and raised. She has completed mission work in Africa, Guatemala, Honduras and Mexico City, focusing on alleviating child malnutrition and hunger. Her greatest passion is to help others discover nourishment and guide them toward a positive relationship with food.

She has worked as a Cardiovascular Nutrition Educator and international speaker for the Miami Cardiac & Vascular Institute at Baptist Hospital South Florida. She is a food and nutrition expert with a proven track record for patient, clinical education for companies such as *Berkeley HeartLab* and *GlaxoSmith Kline/ Inventiv Health*.

A co-author of *The Empty Cup Runneth Over*, *Miami Breast Cancer Experts*, and *Experts in Pink*, Sabrina has appeared on ABC, NBC News, Telemundo, Univision and WLRN-TV. She is currently in private practice at Scientific Nutrition, specializing in all areas of Medical Nutrition Therapy including bariatric nutrition. Sabrina promotes a healthy lifestyle through education and the promotion of organic superfoods under the brand of #QueFlaca, Fuerte & Feliz.

15

OBESITY AND BREAST CANCER

MOISES JACOBS, M.D. AND ALEX FAGENSON, M.D.

Results from the 2007-2008 National Health and Nutrition Examination Survey (NHANES) showed that 68% of United States adults age twenty and older are overweight and obese. This number is up 12% from the early 1990s and the trend is similar with respect to children. This places a significant burden on the health industry. We have learned over the years that being obese puts an individual at increased risk for a multitude of chronic diseases including but not limited to: high blood pressure, joint problems, type 2 diabetes, heart disease, stroke, gallbladder disease, and some cancers. In recent years, it has been shown that there is a direct correlation between obesity and breast cancer (1).

Women who are overweight or obese after menopause have a 30-60% higher chance of getting breast cancer than their counterparts who are lean (2). Many studies have shown that being obese is associated with an increased risk of postmenopausal breast cancer (3). The relationship between obesity and breast cancer may be influenced by the age at which the woman gains weight and becomes obese. After menopause the ovaries shut down and no longer produce estrogen, and at this point the main producer of estrogen becomes fat tissue. As we know, excess estrogen directly aids breast cancer in its growth and thus the more obese you are, the more estrogen you will produce. Additionally, obese people are in a state of ongoing, low-level inflammation that further increases their risk for development of cancer (4). The relationship between obesity and breast cancer may also vary by race; this is currently under investigation.

Thus, it has been proposed that weight loss can help reduce the risk of breast cancer, especially once a woman has gone through menopause. One study showed that women who lost four to eleven pounds after menopause had more than 20% lower risk of breast cancer when compared to women whose weight did not change (5). Weight loss during pre-menopausal years should also have a similar impact with respect to reducing the risk of getting breast cancer; therefore, efforts to achieving a normal body weight should be the goal for all women. With obesity being such a problem, there has been a shift in thought to get the weight corrected as early as possible to avoid breast cancer and all the other negative health effects. Weight loss surgery becomes the best option for a woman once all diet and exercise regiments have failed.

There are currently two major weight loss surgeries offered by surgeons today. Known as the Roux-en-Y Gastric Bypass and the Sleeve Gastrectomy, both are minimally invasive. The Roux-En-Y is the older surgery and the first to become available. This surgery is a two-step procedure with the first being a restrictive phase to create a gastric pouch that reduces the size of your stomach. The second phase is known as the malabsorptive phase and this is where the term bypass comes into play. The surgeon reconnects the small intestine to the gastric pouch in a manner that shortens the distance the food travels. In doing so, the food no longer has the same distance to travel and thus fat and excess calories cannot get fully absorbed. In summary, this surgery creates a smaller stomach, so the patient cannot eat as much, and the food that one eats doesn't get totally absorbed. However, there are many accompanying complications – the most common being deficiencies in key vitamins and nutrients simply because the body does not have enough time to absorb these essential factors. This requires the patient to take many supplements for the rest of their life, increasing the cost of life as well as putting the patient at risk of complications from a lack of satisfactory levels of the essential nutrients. Aside from deficiencies, the patient is at increased risk for constipation, diarrhea, nausea, bowel obstruction, and leaks from any of the connection sites of which there are three. All the long-term complications from this surgery prompted surgeons to come up with a solution that resulted in a procedure known as the Sleeve Gastrectomy.

The Sleeve Gastrectomy is a one-step procedure that only consists of the restriction phase. The surgeon simply cuts the stomach in half, reducing the size of the stomach and quantity of food one can take in at any given time. The surgery is much shorter, straightforward, and carries less long-term complications. Since the surgeon is not reconnecting the small intestine, there is a much less risk of becoming deficient in the essential nutrients. Additionally, since there is only one section that is cut, there is a significantly decreased chance of any leaks, unlike the Roux-en-Y Gastric Bypass, which potentially has three sites that can leak. The time in the hospital after surgery is reduced with the Sleeve Gastrectomy and the patient no longer needs to spend all the money on the vitamins and nutrients that one would need to if they had the Roux-en-Y Gastric Bypass.

In conclusion, weight loss in an obese woman can reduce the risk of breast cancer. It is essential for women to maintain a healthy body weight and those who cannot should seek the option of weight loss surgery to prevent cancer and other long-term health problems. Of the surgeries available, the Sleeve Gastrectomy provides the patient with a simple procedure with minimal risks. This surgery has been adapted from the older technique of the Roux-en-Y Gastric Bypass that has many medical complications and increased financial burden on the patient in the long run.

Dr. Moises Jacobs would like to acknowledge Alex Fagenson, M.D., who was a fourth-year medical student at Florida International University when this chapter was written, for his assistance.

References

1. Nelson HD, Zakher B, Cantor A, et al. Risk factors for breast cancer for women aged 40 to 49 years: a systematic review and meta-analysis. Ann Intern Med. 156(9):635-48, 2012.
2. Huang Z, Hankinson SE, Colditz GA, et al. Dual effects of weight and weight gain on breast cancer risk. JAMA. 278: 1407-11, 1997.
3. Reeves GK, Pirie K, Beral V, Green J, Spencer E, Bull D. Cancer incidence and mortality in relation to body mass index in the Million Women Study: cohort study. BMJ. 335(7630):1134, 2007.
4. Key TJ, Appleby PN, Reeves GK, et al. for the Endogenous Hormones and Breast Cancer Collaborative Group. Circulating sex hormones and breast cancer risk factors in postmenopausal women: reanalysis of 13 studies. Br J Cancer. 105(5):709-22, 2011.

∽

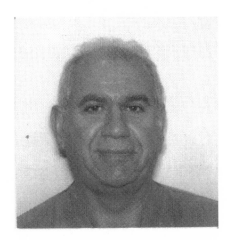

Moises Jacobs, M.D., F.A.C.S. from the University of Miami Medical School in 1979 and finished his general surgery residency at University of Miami/Jackson Memorial Hospital in 1984. He has been performing advanced laparoscopic procedures since 1990 and is credited with performing the first laparoscopic colectomy in 1990. Dr Jacobs is world renowned as a pioneer in laparoscopy and has taught and mentored hundreds of surgeons throughout the world. In addition, he hosts a biannual "minimally invasive" conference where the latest and most innovative surgical techniques in laparoscopic bariatric surgery are presented by the world's experts. Dr. Jacobs has published several research articles and textbooks and has been awarded Unites States patents for his innovative surgical instruments.

Learn more about Dr. Jacobs at his website, www.gastricsleevecenter.com.

16

WHAT DO WE KNOW ABOUT EXERCISE AND YOUR HEALTH?

DON TOROK, PH.D., F.A.C.S.M.

GENERAL GUIDELINES: QUALITY OF LIFE

There are many factors that influence an individual's overall health. It is important to realize that our health is not just physical, but also has components that relate to our mental and social well-being. The crucial role that exercise plays in our overall health profile has expanded and gained greater credence over the years. We know that regular exercise is associated with many positive health outcomes. It wasn't until the 1990's that physical inactivity was identified by both the American Heart Association as a risk factor for heart disease and targeted by the American Cancer Society as preventive action measure.

While we understand that individuals are genetically different, there are some common risk factors everyone should be aware of; these are the things we can control in our daily lives. Here are some healthy habits you can adopt to help reduce your cancer risk:

1. Don't use tobacco products;
2. Limit inactivity;

3. Maintain a normal body weight;
4. Eat a healthy diet.

The American Cancer Society indicates that about one-third of cancer deaths are associated with tobacco use and another one-third of cancer deaths are tied to our diet and activity levels, which is also linked to our body weight (1). Making an effort to address these areas will not only reduce your cancer risk, but will also reduce your risk of developing cardiovascular and metabolic disease.

Let us look more closely at each of these areas and see what we can do to make a positive difference in our lives. The first one seems pretty clear: don't use any tobacco products. This includes cigarettes, cigars, pipes, hookah, chewing tobacco, snuff, blunts, cigarillos, bidis, electronic cigarettes, and other products containing tobacco. There are over 7000 chemicals in tobacco smoke and at least 70 that are known to cause cancer (2).

Be physically active – that is, engage in a minimum of 150 minutes of moderate intensity activity each week (in bouts of at least 10 minutes) with an additional 2 to 3 resistance training sessions/week (8-10 exercises of 10-15 repetitions per set, involving major muscle groups; avoid heavy lifting) and some flexibility or stretching exercises (3-4). The key here is to avoid inactivity. Many individuals revert to inactivity after diagnosis or treatments begins and this may result in the loss of muscle mass, decreases in fitness levels, and increases in body fat and other metabolic (Type 2 diabetes) problems.

Maintaining a normal body weight is in general terms having a normal BMI (body mass index-an index of ones weight in kilograms divided by the square of ones height in meters). There are many body mass calculators online, where you can input you numbers and get your calculated BMI (5). A normal BMI would be between 18.5 and 24.9. Anything below is considered underweight and anything over is considered overweight. Because being overweight is a cancer risk factor and a growing number of Americans' qualify as being over-weight or obese, there is a real need to address our food selections and quantities, in addition to our level of daily activity. It is important to eat a diet that is high in fruits, vegetables, and whole grains, and avoid alcohol (limit one drink/day for women and not more than 2 drinks/day for men) and consume adequate water to remain hydrated.

Why Exercise?

Exercise is a free pharmacological aid available to everyone provided we engage in regular, sustained (at least 10 minute bouts) activity – preferably on a daily basis. Exercise has been shown to assist with improving fatigue, fitness, muscle mass, flexibility, appetite, and quality of life, while reducing depression and anxiety (6, 7). Studies have shown that regular physical activity may reduce the risk for breast, colon, and prostate cancer. As stated above, there are benefits to exercise done during treatment and there are additional benefits from regular physical activity after treatments have been completed. With all this in mind, let us examine how to best put our exercise program together.

Getting Started

As with any exercise program, it is always best to talk with your doctor to just be sure that there are no special concerns that you need to be aware of in planning your activities. Here are some of the factors to consider when you begin your exercise program and some special considerations for some types of cancers.

First, we need to know your present treatment status (before treatment, during treatment, or post treatment). Each of these conditions may require some modifications to the intensity and duration of your daily bouts and will be influenced by your prior exercise history. Always begin at a level where you can be successful and select activities that you find enjoyable. For additional support and encouragement, having an exercise partner adds immediate accountability.

There may be times during treatment, where you may need to cut back or give yourself a little more recovery time. Keep in mind that your exercise program may just be that needed physical release to take your mind off your treatment and experience a good psychological boost. Even after your treatments are over, you may have some lingering side effects that may take some time to diminish. It will be important to keep your program going and to look at the specific aspects of your health that will continue to help improve your quality of life.

General precautions for some groups:

There are certain circumstances where special considerations need to be advised for some individuals (11).

Condition	Precaution
a) Severe anemia	Delay exercise until anemia is improved
b) compromised immune levels	Avoid public areas and pools until immune levels have returned to safe levels
c) severe fatigue	Limit activity to 10 minutes of light exercise until fatigue has improved
d) undergoing radiation	Avoid exposure to chlorine
e) indwell catheter or feeding tube	Avoid pools and other bodies of water where exposure may result in infections and be careful with resistance training of muscle groups that contain the catheter or feeding tube
f) significant peripheral neuropathies or lack of voluntary coordination of muscle movements	Consider exercise equipment that provides more stability (recumbent bike, rowing machine, elliptical machine). Consider supervision during activity.
g) multiple or uncontrolled comorbidities	Consult your physician for advice

Types And Duration Of Exercise

One should start with 10 to 15 minutes of aerobic (walking, biking, swimming, rowing, dancing, etc) activity if you have been sedentary and build up to 30 minutes or more per day. If balance is an issue, you can use a stationary bike or rowing machine. For those individuals that have been exercising, getting more vigorous exercise is fine as long as you do not overdo it to the point that you are still feeling fatigued the next day.

Getting some daily stretching or yoga and two or three session of weight training will help to maintain or build some muscle mass. Stay away from heavy weights and keep the reps to 15 to 20 per exercise for the major muscle groups of the body. Make an effort to record your activity with either a simple diary or use one of the fitness bands or pedometers. Reward your achievements and recognize that it is not a race for today, but a journey into the future. It is the constant small steps that we take each and every day that will help us reach our destination.

Here are some specific considerations that have been linked with exercise and different types of cancer:

Type of Cancer	What we know	Special Considerations
Breast Cancer	a) more fit have lower risk by 20 to 80% (8-9) b) normal BMI and regular physical activity has lower risk of breast cancer. c) 30-60 minutes of moderate to vigorous daily exercise has lower risk of breast cancer.	a) Individual experiencing lymphedema should consider using appropriate compression garments and consult with their physician. b) Individual who had axillary lymph node dissection should refrain from upper body resistance exercises until given approval from their physician. c) Be aware of the risk for fractures for those treated with hormonal therapy or osteoporosis
Colon Cancer	a) more active have lower risk of colon cancer. b) 30-60 minutes of daily moderate to vigorous exercise may protect against colon cancer (8-9).	a) Avoid exercises that create excessive intra-abdominal pressure.
Endometrial Cancer	a) more active have lower risk by 20-40% (8)	a) Avoid exercises that create excessive intra-abdominal pressure until healed.
Lung Cancer	a) more active have lower risk by about 20% (8)	a) start slowly and be sure that the duration and intensity is tolerable for the individual.
Prostate Cancer	a) some evidence that regular vigorous exercise in older men (>65) may slow the progression of prostate cancer(10).	a) Be aware of the risk for fractures for those treated with androgen deprivation therapy (ADT) or osteoporosis

Even though you may do all the "right things," there's always the possibility that cancer may strike. *How are you going to strike back and regain your quality of life?*

A crucial part of establishing a positive outlook is the knowledge that not every day is going to be like past times. What are some of the possible symptoms you may experience during your cancer treatment? It's not uncommon for individuals to deal with the following:

- Depression
- Anxiety
- Body image concerns
- Decreases in self-esteem and quality of life
- Difficulty sleeping
- Muscle weakness

- Weight loss
- Muscle loss
- Loss of aerobic fitness
- Nausea
- Vomiting
- Fatigue
- Pain

Exercise has been shown to assist with improving fatigue, fitness, muscle mass, flexibility, and quality of life while reducing depression (9, 10).

While the benefits of regular exercise are well documented, it's important to remember that there will be days when you'll have to adjust your individual program depending on how you feel. Realize that on any given day you may have to do a little less. The foundation of your exercise routine should be geared to a moderate intensity level and include both flexibility and resistance training.

Since cancer sites and treatments vary, it's critical to seek out an experienced professional to guide your program. While your tailored exercise program is good for your mind and body, it only works if you stick to it consistently. If at all possible, exercise with a buddy or in a group to help you maintain your motivation and adherence to the program.

When you include exercise as part of your daily activities throughout your life, you'll experience both mental and physical benefits. Think of exercise as your own special prescription for mind and body; each and every step you take will help you get closer to your goal of overall wellbeing.

References

1. Nutrition and physical activity guidelines for cancer survivors. CA Cancer J Clin, 2012; 62:242-274.

2. U.S. Department of Health & Human Services: (July 31, 2015) Smoked Tobacco Products. Retrieved from: http://betobaccofree.hhs.gov/about-tobacco/Smoked-Tobacco-Products/

3. Schmitz KH, Courneya KS, Matthews C, et al; American College of Sports Medicine. American College of Sports Medicine roundtable on exercise guidelines for cancer survivors. Med Sci Sports Exerc. 2010; 42:1409-1426.

4. US Department of Health and Human Services. Physical Activity Guidelines for Americans. Washington, DC: US Department of Health and Human Services; 2008.

5. Centers for Disease Control and Prevention: (August 3, 2015) Body Mass Index. Retrieved from: http://www.cdc.gov/healthyweight/assessing/bmi/.

6. Courneya KS, Keats MR, Turner AR. Physical exercise and quality of life in cancer patients following high dose chemotherapy and autologous bone marrow transplantation. Psychooncology 9:127-136, 2000.

7. Courneya KS, Friedenreich CM. Physical exercise and quality of life following cancer diagnosis: A literature review. Am Behav Med 21:171-179, 1999.

8. Lee I, Oguma Y. Physical activity. In: Schottenfeld D, Fraumeni JF, editors. Cancer Epidemiology and Prevention. 3rd ed. New York: Oxford University Press, 2006.

9. McTiernan A, editor. Cancer Prevention and Management Through Exercise and Weight Control. Boca Raton: Taylor & Francis Group, LLC, 2006.

10. Giovannucci EL, Liu Y, Leitzmann MF, Stampfer MJ, Willett WC. A prospective study of physical activity and incident and fatal prostate cancer. Archives of Internal Medicine2005; 165(9):1005–1010.

11. Rock et al., Nutrition and physical activity guidelines for cancer survivors. CA Cancer J Clin, 2012; 62:242-274.

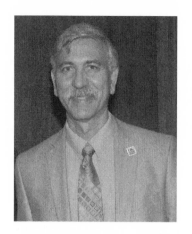

Don Torok, Ph.D., FACSM is an exercise physiologist and fellow of the American College of Sports Medicine. He completed his MS in Exercise Science at Miami of Ohio and his Ph.D. in Exercise Physiology at the University of Tennessee in Knoxville. After receiving his degree in Knoxville, he spent almost two years at the Health Science Center of the University of Tennessee in Memphis before relocating to Florida to accept a position at Florida Atlantic University (FAU). While at FAU, he has been a faculty member, Department Chair of the Exercise Science and Health Promotion, and for the last nine years, Associate Dean of the College of Education.

Don is presently Chair of the Professional Education Committee for the American College of Sports Medicine, on the Executive Committee of the Southeast American College of Sports Medicine, Chair of the South Florida Asthma Consortium, and former Chair of the Tobacco-Free Partnership of Broward County.

17

THE HEALING BENEFITS OF YOGA AND MEDITATION DURING AND AFTER BREAST CANCER TREATMENT

TAMERA ANDERSON HANNA, L.M.C.

What are we learning about Yoga as a support to individuals with breast cancer and cancer in general? Beyond being trendy, Yoga offers many health benefits for both mind and body. However, it is also important to consider what *type* of Yoga is appropriate following a breast cancer diagnosis. In this chapter, I'll share my perspective as a Registered Yoga Teacher who has been trained and certified specifically as a Yoga 4 Cancer (Y4C) teacher, and as a breast cancer survivor with experience in modifying my own practice during my healing.

While there are many forms and variations of Yoga classes available, I will refer here to the benefits found in classes led by Registered Yoga Teachers designed exclusively for individuals healing from cancer. First, an important consideration: following a cancer diagnosis, certain types of Yoga may be contraindicated for conditions such as lymphedema; that's why finding an instructor with some experience and knowledge of how to work with various medical conditions helps ensure the best experience possible – including the discovery of Yoga poses that support healing, treatments, and recovery.

This does not prohibit you from someday returning to or trying out other types of Yoga, for example, a traditional Vinyasa Yoga class, but it's vital to understand your limitations (if you have any) and build up to classes that support your health long-term. If you are unable to locate a class for cancer survivors, it is appropriate to ask an instructor about their experience in working with any conditions that may require modifications for you. If they are not qualified, they can be expected to point you in the direction of a class or instructor more suited to your needs as you heal and undergo cancer-related treatments. Additionally, if you wear a compression sleeve when active, check with your medical doctor as many recommended wearing the sleeve during class.

Prior to beginning any exercise routine, please take treatments such as chemotherapy and reconstruction into account and get approval from a physician familiar with your current medical condition. This applies to post-surgery exercise, and any exercise you engage in while undergoing treatment. Once approved by your doctor, Yoga can be a supportive tool not just for your physical recovery, but for your mental well-being. Depending on the type of Yoga, it can even offer cardiovascular benefits. As a Licensed Mental Health Counselor and Certified Addiction and Rehabilitation Counselor, I often refer individuals to Yoga and meditation in lieu of, or in coordination with group or individual counseling for conditions such as anxiety, grief, depression, post-traumatic stress disorder (PTSD), and pain management, among others.

Yoga offers many medical benefits that impact:

- Mood and Mental Clarity
- Healing and a Sense of Calm (via breathing techniques)
- Range of Motion (a struggle for those who have undergone a mastectomy and lymph node removal)
- Support for Bone Loss (secondary to some treatments like chemotherapy)
- Energy and Stress Levels (which may be diminished from changes in routine and medications)

- Body Weight (weight gain during treatment is not uncommon)
- Lymphedema
- Other Side Effects Like Constipation (alleviated with specific poses)

To sum it up, Yoga counterbalances the impact of cancer and related treatments and assists in keeping the body and immune system healthy. It aids in the prevention of or ability to cope with anxiety; fears about the future; depression-related symptoms associated with diagnosis; grief related to loss of a body part; the *scan-xiety* that results from undergoing multiple tests before, during, and after treatment; or other cancer-induced losses and fears. I have experienced and written about some of these benefits for resources like *Cure Magazine.*

While Yoga does not make your concerns vanish as if by magic, breathing and focusing on living in the moment can help you embrace your days in the best way possible, while releasing what you can't control. Including Yoga in your exercise regimen helps you to get your body moving and promotes the release of chemicals that produce natural endorphins – our happy chemicals. By learning supportive and comfortable breathing techniques, you can help decrease feelings of stress and anxiety, removing your body from the fight-or-flight response.

As you work on learning to live life with and beyond cancer, Yoga can help you with choices that may include ways to further improve your health through diet and exercise. Positive life choices help in managing or reducing the chances of a recurrence. *How and why you ask?* Yoga helps you manage your weight and reduce stress levels your body, both of which can help to minimize risks even after diagnosis. According to the American Cancer Society, obesity is linked to an increased risk for several cancers, including breast cancer, along with heart disease and diabetes (both of which are on the rise). Therefore, exercise is beneficial not only for decreasing the risk of recurrence, but also for general health and wellbeing.

If you are coping with cancer and cancer-related symptoms, Yoga can help you learn to manage feelings of distress or loss; it can also provide support later in life when facing other challenges, along with maintaining your day-to-day health and well-being. In many cases, Yoga provides a sense of support and community when attending a group class. A common theme in Yoga is that there is no competition: you find a pose and practice as it relates to *your* body. This feeling promotes self-acceptance when you may be experiencing symptoms like hair loss; weight gain or weight loss; and maybe even the loss of a body part.

Grief is a common experience with breast cancer; Yoga can help with the adjustments you are making to your body as you practice mindfulness and learn to tolerate the moment. This is done by coming back to your breath and finding the gratitude which also exists concurrently with any grief one may experience. Yoga and group classes can provide a feeling of self-confidence; outside support; and a common, safe place to experience acceptance and understanding of self-care, while promoting healing and recovery.

This feeling of safety can also benefit those who are experiencing symptoms of PTSD because the body does not differentiate between a present stressor or past stressor from years, days, or months ago. What does help is learning how to manage the experience and sensations associated with feelings of PTSD, so the body can begin to find a way to successfully process feelings of trauma -- not just hold it in the body waiting for the next experience. While PTSD may not be cured, learning to breathe effectively and practicing poses can help to lessen the intensity of the experience. Yoga and supportive breathing can teach individuals how to support their mind and body when having a negative experience. For example, many individuals can relate to feelings of anxiety prior to a scan; practicing Yoga helps to reduce anxiety and symptoms of PTSD. Clearing the mind, decreasing stress, and moving the body provide energy and aid in combating fatigue, which is often a byproduct of the healing process. Fatigue is sometimes worsened by cancer-fighting medications and secondary conditions associated with treatments.

Meditation may also be part of a Yoga class or something you can benefit from on its own. The part of Yoga that focuses on Pranayama teaches about the benefits of effective breathing. Thankfully, due to the brainstem we don't have to remind ourselves to breathe...or do we? When we are stressed or feeling anxious, we are most likely *not* breathing effectively. Of course, we are breathing; however, if we focus on where our breath is going, it likely contributes to the basic fight-or-flight response, which means we are potentially breathing into our upper chest or breathing rapidly – which does not help to calm and comfort our bodies.

Breathing rapidly, unevenly, or ineffectively can send a signal our brain that there is something wrong, causing our body and brain to respond to a perceived threat. This perceived threat puts our body into a state of high alert designed to protect us when we need to respond to a dangerous situation. However, if triggered often enough or for a long enough period, the fight-or-flight response can wear down and weaken our immune system. When feeling anxious, fearful, or angry it is harder to think rationally and make good choices. When we learn to meditate and to breathe properly, we can bring our body back to a state of relaxation that supports our immune system and our ability to think clearly and make better choices when presented with a stressful situation. Practicing Yoga or meditation teaches us to focus on the quality of our breathing. Yes, we can breathe without mindfully thinking about it, but choosing supportive breathing and meditation is comparable to eating nutritious foods for the body – and not simply eating to satisfy hunger. What I am saying is, we need to breathe, but we can selectively choose to breathe in a healthy manner. Meditation supports this effort.

When diagnosed with cancer, at first all you might be able to do is breathe, but as I have mentioned it is important to breathe effectively. I particularly enjoy teaching pre-surgery and post-surgery clients to work on their breathing. If you are unable to take a deep breath due to pain, simply learning to breathe in slowly and exhale slowly as comfortably as possible can help send a signal to your brain and the rest of your body to relax. Breathing calmly, for example, stops the release of adrenalin and norepinephrine which are responsible for the body's fight-or-flight sensation. Proper breathing also helps us to begin the process of moving lymph fluid. This in turn, supports our immune system as we allow for increased blood flow to our body and begin to release tension – thereby promoting healing and lessening the sensation of pain. I often compare the resetting of breathing to resetting a computer. Both the body and a computer sometimes need a little help to function better; by rebooting the system, everything falls back into place to run smoothly.

Meditation is also good for enhancing memory, concentration, and combating feelings of mental and physical fatigue, which as I mentioned, can be a side effect from certain treatments. Even a short meditation of as little as five-to-ten minutes can feel as good as a nap and easily practiced while in a hospital setting, during a treatment, at home, or in the office, if returning to work. Fortunately, we now see the trend of practicing meditation and Yoga in the workplace – an excellent way to bring a healthy habit cultivated during healing to your everyday life beyond cancer.

Meditation comes in many styles. That is, there are many ways to meditate and it doesn't have to be complicated. You might find resources from a Yoga or meditation teacher, or possibly from an app on your phone while healing. However, if you find it helpful, I encourage you to explore ways to enhance your practice by trying assorted types of meditation in a group session, provided you inquire about the setting to ensure it is supportive. Early on, while breathing is strained, you might need a simple, seated meditation or one where you can lay down if that is all your body can tolerate. The good news is research is beginning to support meditation as having health bene-fits for mind and body, due to its effectiveness in enhancing the body's ability to relax and decrease inflammation.

Some promising research is being done in places such as the University of Calgary. One study conducted there found that telomeres – believed to be involved in disease and cellular aging – were preserved in those who practiced meditation. When beginning a meditation practice, please exercise caution. It is not uncommon to experience some dizziness early on. Practice at a time and place where you can be monitored or come back to a state of alertness slowly without being rushed. Your blood pressure responds to your body relaxing, and some individuals need to get used to the feeling and practice of meditation. My suggestion is to practice as often as possible – as often as you can tolerate. Some studies and research suggest a practice of as little as three minutes or more a day might be more effective than practicing only once a week. Benefits of meditation are beginning to suggest the reduction in stress associated with the practice assists in supporting immune system function, reducing inflammation in the body, and supporting or slowing the rate of cellular aging. You can find many practices in person or online. I have also written a simple meditation for pain management, which I welcome you to try. Published online with Cure Magazine, it is entitled *Learning to Meditate: A Sample Healing Meditation*.

If you have had surgery for breast cancer, you can begin Yoga once your incisions heal and you are cleared by your medical professional. A supportive Y4C class with its affiliated Yoga poses can assist in helping you adjust to your new body post-surgery, or as you are in early treatments prior to surgery. The Yoga poses done early on in a session typically focus on mindful breathing, warming up the body, stretching the muscles, and assisting with regaining range of motion. Range of motion, scar tissue, and lymphedema are all conditions you want to address and be aware of, depending on the procedures you have experienced. Those who undergo a mastectomy are more likely to have lost range of motion. For anyone who has had lymph nodes removed, be aware of regaining strength and range of motion, but also alert to any symptoms of lymphedema. As a precaution, and while undergoing evaluation for any symptoms for lymphedema, you might be guided to practice poses that help move the lymphatic system in more supportive manner than those outside of a Y4C or cancer-minded class. Movement and Yoga exercises help to get the lymphatic system moving, which consequently supports the immune system and assists in detoxification. Some of the poses in Y4C that help restore the lymphatic system and range of motion, along with strength and flexibility include "Cactus Clap" and "Dirty T-Shirt" among others.

Bone loss and weight management can be negatively impacted by fatigue and the effects of chemotherapy or steroids in the body. Yoga gets the body and brain moving and helps to regulate weight management. Breathing alone helps to refresh the brain, but the postures and poses in an active Yoga class designed for cancer patients helps to preserve muscle strength, which supports the bones. Exercise and movement also promote bone growth and density, which is why some of these Yoga classes include weight-bearing exercise their curriculum.

Movement of the body helps to condition and strengthen muscles and increase flexibility. When your body is made to work, you activate your body and bones to maintain development and support the job of the osteoblasts that build and maintain bone density. You can find support in a class that focuses on poses and movements that assist with balance, along with a modified Vinyasa, for example. In a supportive Yoga for cancer class, several blocks are used to bring the ground to the person; therefore, participants move but avoid extremes found in a traditional Vinyasa class which would likely put too much strain on the body. This is crucial for a patient undergoing cancer treatments or recovering from recent surgery, because it prevents them from putting all their weight into their arms or the core of the body. Using blocks in a practice also supports neuropathy, a condition some individuals develop in their fingers and toes after treatment. It is a nice feeling to be able to exercise and some of the poses offered in a supportive class allow for the weight to be taken off the impacted foot or hand for at least a few minutes.

Constipation is another troubling side-effect from certain treatments, pain medications, changes in diet, and decreased activity. As you get up and begin moving, you can help alleviate the constipation. Furthermore, some of the poses in a supportive Yoga class impact the internal organs and thereby assist in relieving pressure and bloating and helping to move the bowels. If you think about ringing out a dish cloth, you ring out water. Yoga helps move and squeeze internal organs and muscles, which helps to return water to the body. This is also why you are encouraged to drink water after Yoga: it replenishes the body and aids in the natural detoxification process associated with exercise. Practicing poses safely, cued by a knowledgeable teacher, can target areas of your body which have been impacted by treatments and surgeries.

Many hospitals, medical offices, and cancer support communities among other agencies, now offer Yoga classes for healing. Again, I encourage you to read the class description and inquire about the poses or class that are best for you. Those that offer the most benefit for the stage of healing you are in, while also considering any side effects you're experiencing. If you are looking for certified Y4C teachers, you can search for one in your hometown at www.y4c.com. The list is growing as more individuals are obtaining certification annually. Some of them are survivors and medical professionals.

If you're attending your first Yoga class, verify that a mat and other equipment is provided. To prepare for class, dress comfortably, bring water, a compression sleeve if you wear one, and an optional towel (you can use it to cover your eyes in a final sunset pose, if you prefer). Another available option is to bring family members to a Y4C class who can benefit from stress management. Particularly if you are still unable to drive, this is an excellent benefit for you and your caregiver(s). Remember, there is no competition and you don't need prior Yoga experience to enjoy a class. Y4C is also open to previvors who have undergone surgery to lessen their risk of developing breast or ovarian cancer. If it is your first Yoga class, arrive early as you will most likely need to sign a medical release form. While this is an annual requirement, as any changes in health occur, you may need to sign more than one release form per year.

It is my sincerest wish that this chapter has opened your eyes to the medical benefits of a Yoga for cancer practice. May you find a practice or activity that continues to enhance your overall process of healing.

References

1. Cancer.org: "Does body weight affect cancer risk?" http://www.cancer.org./cancer/caner-causes/diet-physical-activity/body-weight-and-cancer-risk/effects.html
2. Cancer.org: "Excess body weight: A major health issue in America." http://www.cancer.org/cancer/cancer-causes/diet-physical-activity/body-weight-and-cancer-risk/health-issues.html
3. Cure Today "How Yoga Can Help in the Cancer Recovery Process." http://www.curetoday.com/community/tamera-anderson-hanna/2018/05/how-yoga-can-help-in-th-cancer-recovery-process
4. Cure Today "Learning to Meditate: A Sample Healing Meditation." http://www.curetoday.com/community/tamera-anderson-hanna/2017/12/learning-to-meditate-a-sample-healing-meditation
5. University of Calgary "Study shows clear new evidence for mind-body connection." http://www.ucalgary.ca/utoday/issue/2014-11-04/study-shows-clear-new-evidence-mind-body-connection
6. Prinster, Tari. YOGA For CANCER: A Guide to Managing Side Effects, Boosting Immunity, and Improving Recovery for Cancer Survivors. Rochester, Vermont: Healing Arts Press, 2104. Print

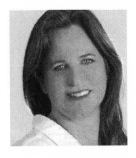

Tamera Anderson-Hanna is a Licensed Mental Health Counselor, Certified Addiction Professional, and Certified Rehabilitation Counselor. She became a Registered Yoga Teacher while coping with breast cancer in 2015. The owner of Wellness, Therapy, & Yoga in Florida where she provides personal wellness services and coaching, Tamera is also a public speaker on wellness-related topics. You can connect with her at www. wellnesstherapyyoga.com.

18

COPING WITH BREAST CANCER

SAMEET KUMAR, PH.D.

A breast cancer diagnosis can present a set of unique challenges for every patient who receives one. No two people will process the experience the same way emotionally; it may be the hinge upon which your life begins to revolve, or it may feel like just a bump in the road. While it's tempting to think there is a "right" way to go through breast cancer, the truth is there are as many pathways as there are people diagnosed. Although each path is unique, there are some commonalities that this chapter will illuminate.

What to Expect From Yourself

For many patients with breast cancer, questions arise in the middle of the night that can seem too difficult to even speak out loud – trying to figure out why you got sick; the statistics you read on the Internet; an off-handed comment your oncologist made – there's no end to the uncertainties your mind can dwell on. Even though most women with breast cancer are living longer and better lives, the hardest questions still have to do with uncertainty and thoughts of death and dying.

Nights like these are quite common for breast cancer patients. If you find yourself pondering these questions over and over, you've probably discovered there are no easy answers. I've come to believe that these are attempts by the mind to try to establish some sense of control amid the ambiguities and uncertainties created by a cancer diagnosis.

The first question most people ask is "Why me?" Even with the best medical knowledge, this is difficult to answer. A perfect storm of genetics, environmental factors, lifestyle, and bad luck does not offer an easy solution, nor does it fit into an easily digested sound bite. Surely, with all of our impressive scientific progress and medical knowledge, there must be a simple explanation?

Unfortunately, not. It seems that the more we learn about breast cancer, the more questions we learn to ask that we didn't know before. Rather than obtain the elusive answers, a much more realistic proposition is to figure out a way to live and thrive with uncertainty. The problem of sickness, suffering, and mortality is one that has been the focus of humanity for millennia. Our current scientific advances seem to have contributed to the mystery instead of solving the riddle. The world's great spiritual traditions have traditionally been used to help us understand the mysteries of our existence. More recently, many popular self-help authors and thinkers have also attempted to answer these questions.

In the popular culture, there's a general belief that cancer can be caused by negative emotions, stressful life events, etc., much like with the flu or heart disease. Research in this area consistently finds that this is not exactly true for cancer, at least not directly.

Many people believe that life's stressful and negative emotions wear down the body's immune system, thereby weakening the ability to fight off cancer cells. Therefore, it is seen as paramount to surround yourself with positive emotions, supportive relationships, and a stress-free lifestyle. These are ideal goals for anyone, with or without cancer. However, as we all know, life is not very predictable, nor is it always pleasant.

Bad feelings, relationships that turn sour, daily stress—these are universal experiences that color all our lives; to place the cause for illness on things over which you have little control over doesn't seem all too helpful. Furthermore, in my experience the belief that stress causes cancer doesn't exactly facilitate relaxation in most people. Stress is inevitable; no one holds the key to turning off that aspect of life in a comprehensive way. I think it's much more helpful to know how to manage stress than to try and pursue an unrealistic life without stress at all.

How Do I Cope?

Over the years, I've observed that people who are involved in their treatment in a deliberate, active way are typically better prepared psychologically for the roller coaster ride that is cancer. However, active involvement means many different things. For some, it means learning all there is to know about breast cancer diagnosis and treatment. For others, it means delegating this knowledge to a caregiver or friend who accompanies them to appointments. For others still, it means focusing on healthy behaviors, or some combination of all of the above.

Although many people find it helpful to research their cancer, not everyone needs to be an expert to be actively involved. Some people choose to become experts in breast cancer; others choose to let their doctors make all the choices, preferring not to know the details. In most instances, you are going to have to decide based on your own comfort level what works best for you. What I frequently tell my patients is to set aside a few hours to learn what you want to know. Generally, the Internet is a decent source of information, but it is frequently discouraging and sometimes irrelevant to your disease variant. Like a local newspaper or the evening news, I've found that generally distressing news about cancer is much more frequent on the Internet than good news. If you find yourself feeling better by learning more about the disease, keep educating yourself. If you find yourself becoming discouraged, demoralized, and depressed, perhaps the information-based approach is not for you. Stick to other areas of self-advocacy, like taking notes during doctor visits, or appointing a willing caregiver as your go-to person for information.

There's one area in which I advise everyone to be equally informed about: pain management. If you are experiencing pain related to your cancer or cancer treatment, it is imperative that you discuss this with your doctor. Adequate and appropriate pain management is the corner stone of psychosocial well-being. If you are in significant physical pain, it will be nearly impossible to do anything else or feel very good until it's under control.

When it comes to emotional pain, most cancer centers utilize a psychosocial team consisting of psychologists, psychiatrists, and/or oncology social workers. You can ask your oncologist's office for guidance in how to connect yourself to these services. Many people also choose to join a support group. In these settings, people of diverse backgrounds and knowledge bases can share feelings and compare notes on their doctors and treatment options. It often feels better to talk to someone who is going through the same thing you are, or has already finished.

Additionally, we now know that not all coping strategies are created equally. The combination of exercise and healthy nutrition can not only help you cope with the stresses of diagnosis, treatment, and uncertainty, it can also reduce the risk of breast cancer recurrence! Studies have shown that women whose breast cancer was hormone- positive face increased risk of recurrence based on alcohol consumption (Zhang et al., 2007). Studies also show that post-menopausal women whose tumors were hormone- negative who exercise more than five times a week can reduce the risk of recurrence by as much as 13% (Peters et al. 2009).

Finally, if you have found that your religious or spiritual beliefs have been helpful to you in the past, use them now. If you are not this type of person, use what has worked before, but only if it promotes health and wellbeing in you and your relationships. You can also explore spiritual teachings that work to help soothe you or give your suffering meaning. Don't hesitate to reach out to close friends or family, or to talk to other survivors. You don't have to go through this alone.

Be Positive or Get Real?

Another prevalent pop culture belief is that being "positive" will aid healing and "negativity" in any form will sabotage your treatment. I find that whenever there is someone talking about how negative emotions can be physically toxic, the atmosphere in the room is decidedly tense – exactly the opposite of what the speaker intended. Similarly, when cancer patients begin to feel that the negativity in their lives has made them sick, this insight generally is accompanied by feelings of guilt, anger, and shame. These are precisely the emotions you are being told to avoid!

In many ways, the pressure to be a positive cancer patient can a self-defeating strategy. Jimmie Holland (2000), one of the pioneers in the field of psycho-oncology, calls this the "tyranny of positive thinking." To sum it up, the journey through cancer, in all its phases ranging from diagnosis to treatment, is likely the most difficult physical – and perhaps also emotional – task that you will ever face. Isn't it unrealistic to force yourself to be the most positive you have been during the most grueling journey of your life? Of course, it always feels better to be hopeful, happy, and driven. But feeling pressured to feel happy rarely results in genuine joy.

The challenge is not to be a positive cancer patient, but an emotionally healthy human being who is experiencing cancer. In my practice over the years, I've found that those individuals who are willing to face their frustrations, anger, shame, guilt—all their very human negativity—are the ones who tend to be happier years later. Denying these essential human emotions and states of mind only stifles the capacity to feel along our emotional and spiritual continuum. Most of us need to experience temporary distress to find a more lasting happiness. The key word here is *temporary*; just as trying to only be happy on positive can be stifling, so to can wallowing in all the frustrations, uncertainties, and misery that cancer can bring.

Remarkably, as yet there is no credible research or evidence to substantiate the idea that the way in which your emotions navigate breast cancer will determine how long you live; to the contrary, research finds that there really isn't an overall effect of how you feel on your long-term health outcome in the face of cancer (Coyne and Tennen, 2010). I find this very liberating to consider; you may experience a ton of pressure to feel one way or the other, e.g. to try to always be positive and grateful. While it may feel better to be positive, it's not always realistic or possible, especially when you're feeling sick or experiencing some painful side effects. Now we can say with some certainty that if you can't feel positive all the time, it really doesn't matter too much in terms of your cancer risk.

Rather than control thoughts and feelings, most psychologists and other mental health practitioners place an increasing importance on accepting them instead as a way to dissolve the power of negative emotions (see Kabat-Zinn, 2005). This approach is in sharp contrast to the repressive, selective attention touted by the "be positive" approach. In my professional experience, repressed feelings don't go away, they just learn to wear masks and re-surface in unexpected areas. Since you can't turn your feelings off, you can give yourself permission to feel them, especially if you know that this is part of a larger process of getting better. Also be re-assured that distress, like any other emotion, tends to be temporary. One of our gifts as human beings the variety of emotions we can feel; we can't feel the good without the bad.

What to Expect From Others

You may have certain expectations of how people around you will react to your illness and you'll quickly learn who's really in your corner. Or you may have already learned this lesson. Don't be surprised if people you had assumed would be there to help seem to disappear, and people whom you'd taken for granted become priceless.

The diagnosis can amplify aspects of relationships, bringing out the best in some and the limitations of others. The happiest breast cancer survivors tend to focus on the relationships that work rather than in disappointment or anger about those that don't. Again, everyone experiences breast cancer differently. There is also a range of how caregivers experience people with breast cancer.

What to Expect in the Future

Most people assume that the day you are told you have cancer is the hardest emotional part of the experience. However, my professional experience tells me that there are three peaks of distress which tend to be universal.

Of course, the first of these is the day of diagnosis. This might be the day your radiologist tells you your mammogram or ultrasound was highly suspicious. It might be when your physician called you to tell you he or she had some unwelcome news to share. It might be the day you felt a strange lump in your breast. Or, it might be when you first met with an oncologist and discussed the specifics of your disease and the treatment options available to you.

Whichever of these examples resonates with your experience, this moment is when you began to grieve the loss of a healthy future. This is not to say that your future won't include health; most of us assume it will. But the day you knew you had cancer, you also learned that this universal assumption is a fantasy. We grieve the loss of that fantasy. I've written extensively elsewhere about how to cope with grief (Kumar, 2005).

The second peak of distress is the day before or the day of your first treatment. This can mean surgery, chemotherapy, or radiation. Whatever treatment modality is indicated for your disease, the day it begins is often filled with a complex mix of anxiety, fear, impatience, and reluctance. Furthermore, if you are receiving steroids like dexamethasone or prednisone as part of your chemotherapy treatment, you may have slept poorly, or feel energized, irritable, or anxious from the medication in addition to the normal stress of treatment. In many ways, the kinds of emotions that emerge on that first treatment day is analogous to the first day of school: deep down, you know this is going to be helpful, but you're reluctant to leave the sheltered, safe, and familiar world behind for this new room full of people you've never met before.

There is no "right" way to feel for these momentous occasions. Truly, the best strategy is to simply get through the day. For many of us, the complex emotions of this first treatment day are fed by another step into the unknown. You wonder what it will be like, how it will feel today and tomorrow, and if it will be like everything you might have heard.

The third peak of distress often occurs shortly after treatment is completed, or shortly before the first follow-up appointment after finishing treatment. Sometimes, there is a peak after treatment is finished, and another one at the three-month or six-month follow-up visit.

You might ask, *"Why would I be distressed about finishing my cancer treatment?"*

I think of the answer to this question as a tendency of our mind to want what is familiar in our lives, no matter what the content of that familiarity might be. When you first started cancer treatment, it may have felt distressing in part because it was new. It felt better as time went on because it became familiar. When you are no longer in treatment, this familiarity to which you've grown accustomed disappears.

Furthermore, when you are receiving treatment, you are actively engaged in a fight against breast cancer. Finishing treatment in many ways can open up issues of uncertainty and vulnerability that you didn't realize were being managed by active treatment. Follow-up visits can only open up this uncertainty by the unexpected news they might bring. It is not uncommon for people to experience increased general symptoms during the week of the follow-up: exhaustion, aches, anxiety, and depression. I am not sharing this with you to help you feel that way. Rather, knowing that this is normal can take quite a bit of the edge off if you should find yourself wrestling with some of these uncomfortable feelings.

What Next?

What do I most hope for when I meet someone with cancer? That they will eventually develop an appreciation for each of life's precious moments after having experienced one its most difficult twists and turns. That is, by experiencing physical illness, you develop an ability to cherish the here-and-now of life's moments rather than dwelling on the failures of the past or the uncertainties of the future. I have found that this focusing on the moment is the only reliable antidote to the unpredictability inherent in human existence. This profound uncertainty about "what if" is at the heart of the fear that most people develop with cancer, or any life-threatening illness.

There are many ways to bring your mind back from the fear and into the reality of today. Many people engage in meditation. I've written a book you might find helpful about how meditation and other techniques can be used to help your mind and body cope with anxiety (Kumar, 2010). Others find artwork to be soothing and comforting. Other people devote more quality time to family and friends. What matters most is not what works for other people, but what works for you. The one thing to remember from the day you are diagnosed is that although you did not choose cancer, you do have choices in how you live, and what you make of the experience.

References

1. Coyne, JC and Tennen, H. (2010). Positive psychology in

cancer care: bad science, exaggerated claims and unproven medicine. *Annals of Behavioral Medicine*, 39, 16-26.

2. Hewitt, M., Herdman, R., and Holland, J. (2004). *Meeting the psychosocial needs of women with breast cancer.* Washington, D.C.: The National Academies Press.

3. Holland, J. and Lewis, S. (2000). The human side of cancer: Living with hope, coping with uncertainty. New York, NY: Harper Collins Publishers, Inc.

4. Kabat-Zinn, J. (2005). *Wherever you go, there you are: Mindfulness meditation in everyday life.* New York, NY: Hyperion Books, Inc.

5. Kumar, S. (2005). *Grieving mindfully: A compassionate and spiritual guide to coping with loss.* Oakland, CA: New Harbinger Publications, Inc.

6. Kumar, S. (2010). *The mindful path through worry and rumination.* Oakland , CA: New Harbinger Publications, Inc.

7. Peters, TM, Schatzkin, A, Gierach, GL, Moore, SC, Lacey, JV, Wareham, NJ, Ekelung, U, Hollenbeck, AR, and Leitzmann, MF. (2009). Physical activity and post-menopausal breast cancer risk in the NIH-AARP diet and health study. *Cancer Epidemiology Biomarkers Prevention*, 18: 289-296.

8. Zhang, SM, Lee, I, Manson, JE, Cook, NR Willet, W., and Buring, JE. (2007). Alcohol consumption and breast cancer risk in the Women's Health Study. *American Journal of Epidemiology*, 165:667–676.

～

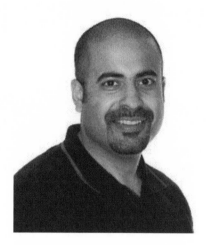

Sameet Kumar, Ph.D., is the clinical psychologist for the Memorial Cancer Institute in Broward County, Florida. He specializes in working with cancer patients and their caregivers. In addition to his training as a psychologist using mindfulness-based therapies, he has also studied with many leading Buddhist and Hindu teachers. He is the author of Grieving Mindfully: A Compassionate and Spiritual Guide to Coping with Loss, The Mindful Path Through Worry and Rumination: Letting Go of Anxious and Depressive Thoughts and Mindfulness for Prolonged Grief.

19

BREAST CANCER AND ITS TREATMENT: EFFECTS ON SEX AND SEXUALITY

CRISTINA POZO-KADERMAN, PH.D.

Breast Cancer and Its Treatment: Effects on Sex and Sexuality

Sex and sexuality are vitally important aspects of being a woman but both are dynamic and change, evolve and are redefined throughout a woman's life and throughout and after her treatment for breast cancer. For a woman with breast cancer, the initial focus of the healthcare team is appropriately on issues related to diagnosis, treatment and management of side effects. The woman herself may be besieged by anxiety and concerns about her survival, her family and many other issues. Sex and sexuality will almost inevitably be affected by breast cancer and its treatments (Table I) but are frequently not discussed early on. Survivors and women undergoing active treatment are encouraged to seek information and express concerns about their sexuality regardless of age, changes brought upon by treatment or their prognosis. Women are treated, not just their cancers, and attention should be given to the whole person.

Sex and women's sexuality are complex and this chapter is not intended to be a comprehensive or exhaustive resource. Rather the aim is to provide information and suggestions based upon concerns often expressed by women with breast cancer.

Table 1. Factors Influencing Sexual Functioning	
• Cancer Treatment	• Pain
—— Surgery	• Changes in body image
—— Chemotherapy	• Relationship factors
—— Radiation Therapy	• Psychological factors
• Other medications	—— Anxiety
• Fatigue	—— Depression
• Stress	

The following will provide a starting point to understand how treatment may affect the sexual aspect of a woman's life (Table 2) and recommendations that may be helpful in adapting to or ameliorating some of these changes.

Table 2. Factors Affecting Sex and Sexuality During Diagnosis, Treatment and Survivorship	
Event	Effect
Pre-diagnosis/Diagnosis	Anxiety*, depression
Surgery	Self-image • Loss or disfigurement of breast • Scarring Diminished sensation in breast Numbness in breast Pain
Radiation Therapy	Changes in skin color Changes in skin texture
Systemic Therapy	Fatigue Alopecia Weight gain Nausea Menopausal changes • Vaginal dryness • Mood changes • Sleep difficulties • Hot flashes
Post-Treatment	Uncertainty Body image Menopausal changes Fatigue Weight gain
*Emotional reactions such as anxiety, may exist to varying degrees throughout and beyond treatment but will generally resolve.	

Defining Terms

Sex and sexuality are distinct but closely inter-related. _Sexuality_ is a _perception of self_ – an identification of one's self as a sexual being and as a woman. It may be expressed in the way a woman talks, dresses, moves and who or what she considers sexually attractive or arousing. _Sex_ is an _act_ that may have many functions: Reproduction, reinforcing relationship bonds and many other outcomes including simply pleasure. Sex may involve a partner or not and can be expressed by touching, kissing, oral sex, intercourse, masturbation and other activities. Women usually experience phases of the sexual response cycle which is comprised of desire (libido), arousal, orgasm and resolution.

Desire is comprised of sexual thoughts and images. In the general population 1 out of 3 women report low sexual desire and 40% of women who go through natural menopause report decreased libido.

Desire is partly mediated by the hormone testosterone. Women produce testosterone in the ovaries and adrenal glands. During menopause there is a reduction in the production of testosterone which may in part impact desire. Arousal or excitement results from sexual thoughts, fantasies and physical touching and stroking. During excitement a woman's heart rate, blood pressure and breathing may increase and there is increased blood flow to the genital areas. The vagina becomes moist, flexible and open, and the body may feel very warm. Arousal is effected in part by psychological, physical, relationship and hormonal variables. For example, hormonal changes during menopause may result in decreased estrogen levels which may cause vaginal dryness and atrophy. This can cause painful sexual intercourse. With enough arousal some, but not all women may reach orgasm during a sexual encounter. Most women need some experience in learning to have an orgasm. Orgasm results in intense pleasure in the genitals as the muscles contract and the nervous system sends waves of pleasure throughout the body. During resolution the body relaxes and gradually your heart and breathing rate decrease. Importantly, it is not necessary for all women to go through all phases to enjoy sexual intimacy.

Sex and Sexuality during Diagnosis Treatment and Survivorship

Pre-Diagnosis and Diagnosis

When a breast abnormality is identified during a self-exam or mammogram, anxiety is expected and normal. Upon diagnosis of breast cancer women often report being emotionally "overwhelmed." Despite this internal turmoil, a woman will need to process a significant amount of often confusing and threatening information and incorporate medical appointments to their already busy lives. Anxiety and fatigue are not uncommon as a woman attempts to balance new stressors with demands from relationships, work and oftentimes children. During this period of time, sex, sexuality and numerous other basic aspects of daily life will likely be disrupted and are not necessarily the focus. Survival is the focus. For those women in relationships, it will also impact their partners.

Local-Regional Treatments

Surgery – whether lumpectomy (partial removal of breast) or mastectomy (complete removal of one or both breasts) – is the primary treatment of early-stage breast cancer. A woman's breasts may have been central to her sense of sexuality/attractiveness and for many women a source of pleasure during sex. A woman may experience post-operative pain/discomfort, scarring and changes in her body image. After complete removal of one or more breast(s) a woman may have loss of sensation or numbness on the chest wall at the mastectomy site. While reconstructive surgery may rebuild the shape and size of the breast, the pleasure from caressing the breast and nipple is likely to be changed, diminished or absent. Over time, women may experience a return of sensation in the reconstructed breast but will not likely be the same as before surgery.

For women undergoing lumpectomy, temporary pain, discomfort or numbness typically resolves over time and typically no long-term effects on sensation are evident. For women undergoing lumpectomy, radiation therapy may also be included as a part of local treatment. As a consequence there may be breast tenderness or pain during treatment which diminishes over time. Some women report a change or decrease in sensitivity. Additionally, there may also be changes in the color and/or texture of the skin and hardening of surgical scars in the irradiated area. While women who preserve their breast may have better body image, they do not have better or more sex. Now and throughout treatment, communication with partners will be important and can serve to further reinforce the relationship.

Systemic Therapy

Systemic therapy basically refers to drugs taken orally or received via an infusion at the oncologist's office or cancer center and compromise different types of medicine (Table 3).

Table 3. Types of Systemic Therapy for the Treatment of Cancers		
Type of Therapy	Function	Brand (generic) Examples
Chemotherapy	Kills tumor cells	Adriamycin (doxorubicin), Cytoxan (cyclophosphamide), Taxol (paclitaxel), Taxotere (docetaxel)
Hormonal therapy	Blocks estrogen receptors on tumor cells or decreases estrogen levels	Nolvadex (tamoxifen), Arimidex (anastrozole), Femara (letrozole), Aromasin (exemestane), Faslodex (fulvestrant)
Biologics	Interferes with biologic processes of cells	Ibrance (palbociclib)
Targeted therapy	Affects specific targets believed to drive cancers	Herceptin (trastuzumab), Perjeta (pertuzumab), Kadcyla (T-DM1)

Drugs given after surgery, for early stage breast cancer, are referred to as _adjuvant_ therapy. In the case of chemotherapy this is time-limited and may last a few months; with anti-HER2 trastuzumab treatment it may last up to 1 year; while oral hormonal therapy may be taken daily for 5 or more years. For women with metastatic breast cancer, drug treatments are typically continuous. Each drug has a distinct side-effect profile while also frequently having toxicities in common with other drugs. A comprehensive description of drug side effects is well beyond the scope of this chapter so the focus will be on those which affect a woman's appearance hence her sense of sexuality and those that may interfere with sexual functioning.

Body-Image Changes: Treatment of breast cancer will likely result in certain visible changes to a woman's body (Table 4). For many women the most difficult side effect from some of the chemotherapies used to treat breast cancer is hair loss or alopecia wherein a woman loses the hair on her head, eyebrows, eyelashes and perhaps pubic area.

Table 4. Potential Common Body-Image Changes Associated with Systemic Therapy

- Hair loss
- Weight gain
- Changes in skin tone or texture
- Changes in nail color

For most women, hair is an important part of their sexuality and feelings of attractiveness. Many women with breast cancer state that it is hair loss that is most associated with "looking like a cancer patient." For patients with localized, early-stage breast cancer, hair loss is usually completely reversible after cessation of adjuvant chemotherapy. Emerging evidence supports the use of "cold caps" or "cooling caps" during the administration of chemotherapy to ameliorate scalp hair loss and women receiving chemotherapy are encouraged to discuss this option with their oncologist. Women should be informed beforehand about the likely side effect of hair loss and the option of using wigs, scarves or hats.

Weight gain is common – a further assault on body image– is likely due to multiple factors including normal aging, changes in diet and physical activity during treatment, and hormonal changes caused by treatment. Women receiving tamoxifen often blame this treatment; however, no solid evidence supports tamoxifen as the only culprit and weight gain is likely due to a combination of factors. Other potential effects of chemotherapy on body image which are often reversible after treatment ends may include changes in skin tone and texture or discoloration of fingernails and toenails. Programs from the American Cancer Society like "Look Good, Feel Better" provide helpful strategies to deal with some of these physical changes.

Changes in Sexual Functioning: The most ubiquitous change associated with cancer treatment is fatigue and its impact on sexual functioning is easily appreciated. Women are often tired having to juggle work, family and social responsibilities even before a cancer diagnosis. Sex if not made a priority may take a backseat due to exhaustion. Fatigue during breast cancer treatment has multiple sources including the emotional upheaval associated with a threatening disease and life demands associated with medical appointments and treatment. Fatigue is also associated with many systemic treatments used to treat breast cancer including chemotherapy and hormonal therapies such as tamoxifen which is associated with the development or exacerbation of hot flashes that may disturb sleep and can then result in feeling tired during the day.

Several activities may help to ameliorate fatigue (Table 5). Women will often try to continue their "normal" activities during and after treatment. Learning to pace oneself and accept changes in energy level helps to avoid frustration with setting up unrealistic expectations. Women may keep a diary to track their energy levels and become aware of the peaks and valleys. For example, if energy level is highest in the morning then schedule most important activities early in the day. For example, it may be better to be sexually intimate early in the day than at the end. While it may seem paradoxical, exercise can help increase energy level even walking at a moderate level several times a week. Using relaxation with imagery aimed at recharging your body as well listening to upbeat music and dancing can help combat fatigue and increase sexual feelings.

Table 5. Activities to Reduce Fatigue

- Use a diary to track energy levels, Pacing
- Prioritize demands
- Enlist others to help with daily tasks
- Exercise
- Relaxation
- Meditation/imagery
- Music

The most direct and significant effect of systemic therapy on sexual functioning is due to changes in the hormonal milieu resulting in menopause or a menopause-like state. At menopause, women experience a decline in estrogen which is a natural change for all women and is gradual occurring over several years the average age being 52.

Menopause may be associated with a number of changes (Table 6) including weight gain, hot flashes, night sweats, moodiness and vaginal dryness which can impact sexual functioning. Women will also experience a decline in the "male hormone" testosterone which may be associated with a reduction in libido.

Table 6. Menopausal Symptoms

- Vaginal dryness and decreased elasticity
- Hot flashes
- Sleep difficulties
- Fatigue
- Changes in mood
- Weight gain
- Decreased libido (sexual desire)

In younger women with hormonally sensitive breast cancer medical or surgical treatments that suppress or remove the ovaries will result in an abrupt shift to menopause which may be more difficult than naturally-occurring menopause. Additionally, treatment with certain chemotherapeutic agents particularly alkylating agents like cyclophosphamide may also result in premature menopause. This risk varies based upon the age of the woman at treatment, wherein the risk of premature menopause is 25-40% in women under 40 years old and 76-90% in those over 40. Postmenopausal women receiving hormone replacement (HRT) will be asked to discontinue HRT once diagnosed if their breast cancers are "hormonally driven." Often this will result in a return of some menopausal symptoms. Post-menopausal women are also often treated with aromatase inhibitors (i.e., Arimidex, Femara) which will further decrease circulating estrogen levels.

Among the changes associated with menopause, by far the most important predictor of sexual dissatisfaction is vaginal dryness which may result in pain and even bleeding during intercourse. Several over-the-counter, non-hormonal vaginal moisturizers and lubricants are readily available and if used properly, have been highly successful in countering this particular side effect (Table 7). The first step in combating vaginal dryness is to use a vaginal moisturizer regularly every other night prior to bedtime so the moisturizer can be absorbed while you sleep. The moisturizer is to be used regardless of sexual activity. Even if a woman is not currently in a sexual relationship, vaginal health is important and by using a vaginal moisturizer the vagina stays moist and flexible. There are several moisturizers available such as Luvena or Replens. Some women report that Replens, if used regularly can be as effective as estrogen cream. When sexually active, before penetration a woman needs to use a vaginal lubricant. Common lubricants are Astroglide and K-Y Jelly. It is best for the lubricants to be water-based and to avoid those with perfumes, flavors or parabens which can cause irritation. The lubricant needs to be applied not just inside the vagina but also on the vulva. Women may use the application of lubricant as part of foreplay and include their partner. If vaginal penetration continues more than a few minutes, lubricant may need to be reapplied. Vaginal suppositories which will melt inside the vagina are also good options for some women and can be applied prior to sexual activity. Petroleum jelly, skin lotions and oil-based lubricants are not good choices as they can raise the risk for yeast infections.

Finally it is worthwhile noting that in addition to systemic treatments for breast cancer, a number of other commonly taken medications may also contribute to or exacerbate sexual problems. For example, allergy medications may help dry up nasal membranes but also exacerbate vaginal dryness. Women should check with their physician to determine if any medications they are presently taking have sexual side effects.

Table 7. Interventions for Vaginal Dryness
Nonhormonal and Over-the-Counter

- **Vaginal Moisturizer**
- Use every other night
- Use prior to bedtime
- Use regardless of sexual activity or relationship status
- Commonly used products include Replens (polycarbophil), Luvena, hyaluronic acid

- **Vaginal Lubricant**
- Use prior to penetration and during sexual activity
- Apply inside the vagina as well as on the vulva
- Avoid perfumes, flavors and parabens which may cause irritation
- Commonly used products include: Astroglide, K-Y Jelly or vaginal suppositories

Enhancing Your Sexual Life During and After Breast Cancer Treatment

The most crucial aspect of having a healthy sex life is for women with breast cancer to communicate with their partners. Most partners, if in is a good relationship, will report continued attraction and interest in sex. Partners may not initiate sexual contact for fear of hurting the woman or appearing insensitive in wanting to be sexual. Partners need to be informed on treatment's physical, emotional and sexual possible side effects. Women may want to discuss fears of rejection and other anxieties. Most partners harbor the same concerns and worries. Sharing, listening and keeping communication open are key to a good relationship.

Initially women may not feel ready for sexual activity. Most women enjoy being touched and getting a massage or foot rub which may be an initial step. Women need to communicate if they have pain anywhere in their body and limit touching. When ready for intimacy, women need to make time for it and make sure they are not feeling too tired. The emphasis needs to be on pleasure rather than performance. Create a relaxing environment, light candles and allow time to get "in the mood." Listening to relaxing music, holding hands, kissing and dancing are ways to increase intimacy. Taking a tub bath or showering together are ways to gradually get more comfortable with sharing bodily changes and engage in sensual touching. While treatment may have brought about changes in where and how a woman feels pleasure, exploring alternatives can be approached with a mindset of having fun. Watch an erotic movie or read erotic literature to each other. Go shopping for sex toys. Rediscover the joys of "petting" and take extra time for foreplay. Try oral sex and masturbation with your partner. Experiment with sexual positions. For example, some women may no longer find the missionary position comfortable for sexual intercourse. By changing and being on top, women have more control on the depth of sexual penetration.

Exercise is associated with increased sexual desire and better sexual functioning. Women may also benefit from exploring their bodies and learning what makes them feel good. Self-stimulation, using a vibrator and practicing Kegel exercises, all may help women to better understand their sexuality. Kegel exercises are a way for women to become aware of their vaginal muscles and learn to relax them during sexual activity. Kegel exercises can help alleviate painful sexual intercourse. Once a woman has had painful sexual intercourse she may become tense in sexual situations and may unconsciously tighten the muscles leading into the vagina. Once these muscles tense, penetration becomes more difficult and more painful which then leads to further tension. Learning to relax the vaginal muscles can make penetration easier. In addition, intentional tensing and relaxing vaginal muscles during sexual intercourse can increase sensation and pleasure for both the woman and her partner.

While this chapter has focused on sexuality, it is important to keep sex in perspective. While a woman's sex life may change after breast cancer, intimacy and closeness with her partner may increase.

Couples often feel a sense of gratitude to have survived and a renewed focus on trying to enjoy life to its fullest.

The preceding information obviously applies to women in a relationship with a sexual partner. However for single women, a number of issues will arise beforehand with potential partners including how and when to discuss their history of breast cancer and how it may affect their relationship and sexual life. Other available resources such as the American Cancer Society's "Sexuality for the Woman with Cancer" provide a more thorough coverage of these issues.

Table 8. Tips to Enhance Your Sexual Life During and After Breast Cancer Treatment

- Be patient with yourself and your partner
- Communicate with your partner
- Share what you have learned about how cancer may affect your sex life
- Share your feelings and listen to your partner's fears and concerns
- Discuss your preferences and ask about his/hers
- Emphasize intimacy and pleasure over performance
- Bathing together
- Sensual touching or massage
- Erotic literature or movies
- Extra time for foreplay
- Keep an open mind to alternative ways to experience pleasure
- Sexual positions
- Oral and manual stimulation
- Adult toys
- Exercise
- Kegel exercises

Conclusions

The diagnosis, treatment and survival of breast cancer present numerous physical, psychological and social challenges to a woman. While the primary concerns of survival and quality-of-life are often center stage, it will be important for many women to maintain or reclaim their sense of sexuality and to continue a satisfying sexual life throughout treatment and beyond. Many sexual side effects are reversible after completion of treatment and others may be effectively addressed through relatively straightforward activities of the individual woman, her partner and her healthcare team.

Helpful Resources

1. **Sexuality for the Woman with Cancer** https://www.cancer.org/treatment/treatments-and-side-effects/physical-side-effects/fertility-and-sexual-side-effects/sexuality-for-women-with-cancer.html
2. **Look Good...Feel Better** 1-800-395-LOOK, or visit www.lookgoodfeelbetter.org
3. **International Society for the Study of Women's Sexual Health (ISSWSH)** http://www.isswsh.org/
4. **American Association of Sexuality Educators, Counselors and Therapists (AASECT)** http://aasect.org/

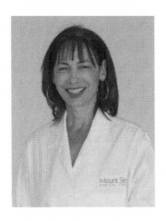

Dr. Pozo-Kaderman received her Ph.D. in clinical psychology at the University of Miami. She completed her internship at Cornell Medical College at New York Hospital and followed with a fellowship in Psycho-Oncology at Memorial Sloan Kettering Cancer Center Psychiatry Department. She started and was the Director of the Psychosocial Oncology Program at the Mount Sinai Cancer Center for 18 years and was also the Administrative Director of Psychosocial Oncology Courtelis Center, Assistant Professor in Psychiatry, at the University of Miami for 2 years. She has been actively involved in training doctoral students in psychosocial oncology. She has published articles in peer reviewed journals primarily on breast cancer. A certified sex therapist, she now works part-time at the Mount Sinai Comprehensive Cancer Center and is adjunct faculty at the University of Miami, Department of Psychology.

20

THROUGH THE EYES OF AN ONCOLOGY NURSE

JANET VILLALOBOS, A.R.N.P

My name is Janet Villalobos. I was the first person in my family to attend college. Today I am a Board Certified Acute Care Nurse Practitioner, working in Pain Management at the University of Miami, Sylvester Comprehensive Cancer Center. There, our practice focuses mainly on cancer pain, which provides for a very rewarding career. There is no limit to the satisfaction I feel from seeing these patients obtain the pain relief they so desperately desire. I consider myself very lucky to have the opportunity to be part of that team.

I began my career in healthcare at Baptist Hospital, where I volunteered my time during my college years and later worked as an emergency room technician. Since then, I've worked as a registered nurse with over 15 years of healthcare experience in different specialty areas including pediatric oncology and ICU nursing, medical/surgical telemetry, home health, case management and adult oncology.

In addition to my extensive clinical background, my academic achievements include two bachelor degrees, one in biology and one in nursing, graduating Magna Cum Laude from Barry University School of Nursing. Throughout my nursing career, I have forged a path which has led me toward helping patients deal with disease. For this reason I felt that a Master's degree in nursing would give me the tools to better serve my patients by integrating the medical model and nursing model.

I am also the mother of a very beautiful 12 year-old daughter who is the light of my life and my reason for living. She has been with me through all the tough times, even when she didn't know it. She is an exceptional human being and a loving child with everyone she inter- acts. She always displays good manners around others and has a very unique quality which I wholeheartedly admire; she is very polite and discreet with others. She makes her mother proud every day.

Nursing was not my first choice. In fact, it wasn't even my second choice, but it was the best one I could have ever made. It has defi- nitely changed my life. As a young girl, I wanted to be a teacher. I knew I wanted to do something that involved children. Don't all kids think alike? My daughter now says the same thing... she would like to be a teacher or a neonatal nurse. It almost always involves working with young ones. Whenever I would tell my mother about my dreams of becoming a teacher, she would reply that it wasn't a good idea because it paid too little; that I wouldn't be able to make a good living as a teacher. The best thing for me to study, she would say, was medicine. After all how many physicians in the United States do you see driving around a beat up car and living in the projects?

Encouragement without guidance led me to enroll as a premed major in college to earn a Bachelor's in Biology. Eventually I wound up in medical school, but because I wasn't part of the elite and just an average student, I ended up attending a foreign medical school. Needless to say, this would not be my calling; in the end the hurdles became too overwhelming so I left medical school to start nursing school. Since I had already been accepted to Barry University School of Nursing, I decided to give that career a shot. Never in my life did I imagine the personal satisfaction I would gain from entering into a field with such immense responsibility and such little appreciation for what one does. You may ask: *How can she obtain gratification from doing something that very few appreciate?*

Trust me, I ask myself the same question at times. Especially on the nights I'd come home after a long shift and felt as if I had left my heart and soul on that unit; I had nothing left inside when I returned to my home. Sometimes I was an empty shell. But then there were those "other" days. I call them "The Glory Days."

Don't get me wrong, I loved medical school and I didn't leave because of academic reasons. I would've finished had circumstances been different.

Nursing school was a breeze compared to medical school, I must admit. I graduated Magna Cum Laude without any effort outside of the classroom; I couldn't wait to finish and get on with my life. When I first graduated from nursing school, I attended an open house at Jackson Memorial Hospital with the hopes of going into ICU nursing, but it didn't go beyond the initial interview. I was discouraged because there was too much red tape.

Then I heard about Miami Children's Hospital hiring graduate nurses. There I interviewed and got hired on the spot as a pediatric oncology nurse. That is how my relationship with oncology started. I was very excited to be able to work with children. I wasn't a teacher, but I was looking forward to interacting with kids and making an impact in their lives. Working with kids in the medical field is quite different from adult nursing. Much of this divergence is due to the parents – to whom I never gave a thought.

When you take care of children, you take care of the entire family. It's like dealing with a gangster who is surrounded by all his body guards or a politician by his advisors! I didn't know what I was getting myself into at the time. I definitely met some beautiful souls there, no doubt. Others were not so beautiful and in fact very difficult to deal with. Throw in the parents and you have a recipe for disaster. I remember one in particular whose port I was trying to access. Both parents and family members were present throughout the entire process. Imagine the pressure to not lose my sterile field, especially having other more experienced nurses critiquing my technique in front of everyone and the child screaming and thrashing about while he was held down.

How do you gain that child's trust after sticking him with a needle? If I missed and had to try again, how would I deal with the vocal disapproval of his angry parents? So here I was, a new nurse, fresh out of school who hadn't yet passed my Boards and already inflicting pain on those little souls I wanted to help. In particular, I remember one incident where a boy spat on my face because I had to re-access his port. While I didn't like what he did, I disliked his punishment even more. With one swift movement his mother slapped him so hard his face swung to the side and back causing him to hit his head against the side rail. It was not a pretty experience, but unfortunately one that I will never forget.

He and I never connected, but I loved that child and he will remain a part of me as long as I live. Not because of that incident – although it has marked me forever – but because he was "special" as his parents would call him. He wasn't a typical nine year-old boy who reasoned and cooperated. He had the mind of a four year-old. Yes, he was mentally challenged but what was sadder than his disability was the fact that his parents had not come to terms with it. They loved their boy but didn't know how to deal with him. Hell, I gotta give it to them, it was hard for *anyone* to deal with him.

But he won my heart because he was sweet when he wasn't fearful due to being poked. During these times, he'd be very affectionate and play endlessly. Sometimes he would sit in his room and sing while he played. That always touched my heart so I would finish my hourly rounding and to-do's before taking off to his room to spend time with him – even if just to watch over him and pray we would be able to cure him. He was one of the lucky ones; he survived cancer and was discharged after just two treatments.

Others didn't fare so well. Death is one aspect of oncology nursing I have never come to terms with. I remember a nine month-old boy with blond hair and blue eyes. He looked like cherub angel. Both his parents were young and he was an only child. It was approximately six months from the time of diagnosis to death. I recall that moment vividly. His father held him in his arms while he fought for breath. He'd lovingly rock him and say "it's okay buddy, it's alright sweetheart." Heart-wrenching.

Writing about it now brings tears to my eyes. More than 50 percent of those children died from cancer during those years. I would meet a new child and his family and fall in love with them only to have the child ripped away from us by this devastating disease. At that time, I couldn't identify what was going on in my head. I dreaded going to work and I would torture myself thinking about those kids and their parents when I wasn't there. I never identified what was happening to me. Although I was an effective nurse who never made mistakes, I demonstrated somewhat aberrant behavior with my colleagues and I didn't get along too well with some parents.

Of course, I never thought about talking about my feelings and worries with anyone; I simply went on day-to-day trying to cope with becoming too attached to the children and then having to say goodbye. I felt that oncology treatments were a failure. *What was the point of putting all these children through hell if they were only going to die in the end?* I remember one mother took me aside and asked me what I would do if I had to make a choice of putting my child through a bone marrow transplant. At first, I tried the usual response. I remained professional, noting that giving her my personal opinion would not be the right thing to do. In response, she broke down and started crying. Since we'd become quite close during the treatments, I had no choice but to be a friend.

After warning her that she had asked me for my sincere advice and that I was going to offer it, she said she would consider whatever I told her. My answer was a resounding NO. I would never put my child through a bone marrow transplant. I had seen what that treatment did to the children and I had not seen one survive in the year I had been a nurse. I said, "If he were my son, I would get him out of here and spend the time he has left doing things he wants to do."

Please understand I was not a parent at the time; I had no idea how protective one becomes with their own child. Back then it was easy for me to decide. After all he was not my son. I regret to say that I'm not so sure anymore what my answer would be to that question. In the end, she put him through the transplant and he did not survive. But had she not attempted to save her child, could she have lived with herself? I look at it as a no-win situation; any decision she took would have been mired in regret.

Although it is doesn't make up for her loss, she had three other children; I was comforted by that to some extent because she'd still have a reason to live. Her other small children still needed her and their father. I also took note of family dynamics. While many families are supportive, others are remarkably dysfunctional. Whenever I encountered these kinds of families I'd wonder, *why in the world did God allow these children to get sick?*

There was a little girl with whom I became especially close. She had leukemia and I remember the first time she came in for her first round of treatment. At the time of diagnosis, she was just nine years-old and led into the unit by her mother and three other siblings. Her mother was a young woman wearing high heels, tight jeans and top and hair extensions, with a face covered in make-up. She was overly bejeweled with thick gold hoop earrings and several gold teeth. Each of her children – including the newly diagnosed angel – was poorly groomed, dressed in clothes about several sizes too small, with wet noses and disheveled hair.

To my dismay, this tiny patient was dropped off and left alone with no spare clothing or shoes. I remember she was too big for the smaller hospital gowns, forcing us to give her adult gowns. She would walk around the unit dragging the gown behind her and bunching it up in her hands in front of her. I made it a point of sharing good times with her and requesting her as my patient whenever she was there. I dreaded going home and leaving her all alone overnight; a helpless, innocent child with no one to dry her tears or hold her through the night to soothe away her fears. She didn't ask for this. She hadn't done anything to deserve her misfortune. Didn't other people see this?

I would observe the other nurses around me and found them so distant from the patients. Some would tell me that I would get used to it eventually. They seemed like business as usual at all times. I wonder if some of them had undergone counseling where they'd learned to deal with the stress and profound sadness that comes from losing a patient. After some more lives loved and lost, I decided I couldn't deal with it anymore and resigned.

Have you ever heard the expression "whoever does not like soup gets two servings?" Well that saying definitely applies to me. I went back into oncology nursing at the University of Miami about five years ago, but this time with adults. As I mentioned earlier, working with adults is definitely different than working with children. Although my heart still goes out to them due to their devastating diagnosis, I have comfort in the knowledge that they have lived already and are, for the most part, fully capable of taking care of themselves and understanding their diagnosis – sometimes even capable of embracing it, accepting it, and fighting it consciously. With the advancement of science in the field of oncology, many patients who once got a death sentence with this diagnosis are now surviving to live another day. With this said, my outlook on the treatments and the diagnosis itself has molded into one of hope for the future; perhaps I can shed some light on this for you if you are battling this tough disease and need some tips.

Getting a cancer diagnosis can be overwhelming. The worst emotion that will probably keep anyone up all night is fear of the unknown. For this reason alone, many patients will not seek medical attention, even when they are aware that their bodies have undergone some kind of change. The best advice I can offer as a nursing professional is for patients to become informed about their diagnosis and treatment options. It is okay to get a second opinion. Often this involves seeking another healthcare provider who can review your records and test results, and confirm the initial diagnosis and treatment or suggest a different approach. New innovative treatments are discovered continuously and a second opinion may also lead to a change in the diagnosis and treatment approach. It may even save your life. Once a cancer diagnosis is received, it is important to make a list identifying important questions like the type of cancer, the specialists able to treat the type of cancer, and the treatment choices available. Another important question to ask involves the effectiveness of one treatment modality over another.

Take for example, breast cancer. Breast cancer types can vary quite extensively. There are many treatments which could be effective in eradicating this disease. In addition to the most common treatments such as surgery, chemotherapy, and radiation, there are more innovative interventions such as targeted therapy and hormone therapy which provide personalized treatment. Breast cancer, like any other type of cancer, has the best chance of being cured if caught in the earliest stages. Knowing the stage of the cancer can shed light on how extensively the cancer has expanded throughout the body, whether to nearby lymph nodes of other organs. This will usually dictate how it is treated.

Knowing the grade of the tumor is also important. The higher the grade, the more likely it is to grow more quickly. The use of hormone therapy will be determined by whether or not the tumor is receptive to estrogen or progesterone. Some breast cancers overproduce a substance called HER2. In these cases, they can be treated with targeted therapy. Once the type of breast cancer is determined, then a treatment plan will be recommended.

So now that you have a cancer diagnosis and a treatment plan, what's next? Once you and your healthcare provider decide which treatment is best for you, getting prepared for what lies ahead is key. Most importantly, you'll need a positive attitude. I have seen patients on both side of this psychological spectrum, and guess who did better? Next, know what to expect after surgery. For women who choose to undergo a mastectomy to avoid the risk of recurrence, there are usually two different approaches to reconstruction.

One approach involves the use of a flap, which is tissue obtained from another part of your body. Another is the use of a tissue expander which slowly expands your breast tissue in order to accommodate an implant which is done with a second surgery. Surgeries times can vary depending on the extent of intervention needed. It can be either an outpatient or inpatient procedure and it may even require you to stay several days in the hospital. You can definitely expect swelling, scarring, and possibly a change in breast sensitivity. Overall recovery can take up to six weeks.

Expect to take pain medication and be sure to ask your surgeon if performing surgery on the natural breast simultaneously with your reconstruction would be a good idea so that both look more symmetrical. Many women fail to think about this and often undergo unnecessary surgeries to get their breasts to look the same. Remember nipple reconstruction too! Working in a cancer inpatient unit, in addition to administering the treatments ordered by providers to our patients, I also dealt with the side effects that often plague these patients, mostly nausea and vomiting, fatigue, neutropenia, and hair loss.

Most breast cancer patients are given chemotherapy and radiation on an outpatient basis, but I can still offer some savvy advice for these patients as they will experience these at home. Prevent nausea and vomiting by eating small, frequent meals consisting of foods you like. Most chemo regimens will change your palate; therefore, the the foods you ate previously might now be unpleasant for you. Drink plenty of fluids in small sips throughout the day instead of trying to chug down a whole glass. For combating fatigue, take advantage of frequent rest periods during the day. Don't do too much at one time.

Maintain regularly scheduled time for physical activity whether walking, light jogging, or even bike riding. Make sure you stay tuned to your inner self with relaxation techniques, yoga, or meditation. For times when you are neutropenic (low white blood cell count/low immune system activity) from the chemotherapy, make sure you practice a good hand-washing technique since this has been known to be the best prevention of infection. If you develop a fever, contact your oncologist right away. You will need immediate hospitalization and antibiotic therapy. Stay away from crowded places, children, and pets while you are neutropenic. Children can carry lots of bugs around from picking toys up off the floor or playing outside and I don't have to explain about dogs who roam around outside in the yard and come into the house without cleaning their feet or washing their hands!

For many women, losing their hair in addition to losing a breast can mean losing their feminine identity. While undergoing treatment, do not use abrasive shampoos or heat styling devices such as blow dryers or flat irons. Also if you know your treatment is going to cause you complete hair loss, give yourself a shorter cut or shave your head completely. If you decide to shave, you can choose different hair coverings from hats and scarves to wigs. You can even buy these before you need them so you are prepared when the time comes. Hair and make up are integral to feeling feminine. You can optimize your look by applying make up to help you feel more like yourself and you can even use a self tanner to combat the pallor that more often than not accompanies cancer treatments. Remember to trim, file and color your nails to cover any discolorations which may result from some chemo treatments. Be sure to do this yourself or have a friend do it with your own tools to avoid getting an infection from shared tools.

Unlike children who are automatically cared for by their parents, grandparents and other family members willingly and without asking for help, many adults isolate themselves from family and friends when faced with a cancer diagnosis. They don't want to overburden their loved ones. But to you I say this: enlist the help of family and friends. Everyone pitching in equally means there is less to do for any one caregiver, providing for adequate time off and a more effective support system. Caregivers should take turns staying with you overnight in the hospital and at home. Take inventory of what each person is good at doing and don't be afraid of asking them for help – from cooking to cleaning, laundering, medication administration, errand running and child care.

No one person should be left to care for someone with cancer by themselves. It can cause something called caregiver burnout and it's not fair to the caregiver – especially if there are others willing to help. I took care of a patient whose daughter stayed with him during the day and whose wife would come in and keep him company overnight. During the weekends, his son-in-law would stay with him while his sister would cook his favorite homemade meals. They worked in sync, each knowing what needed to be done. One day I asked them how they did it. They told me that they'd gotten together when he was first diagnosed, made a list of responsibilities, and divided them up. It worked like a charm! It's important for caregivers to accept help from others and continuously communicate with one another.

At the beginning of this chapter I related that nursing had been the best career choice I ever made. Well if you read this chapter in full, now hopefully you understand why. Oncology nursing is a tough field because it showcases our mortality as human beings and involves giving of oneself as a person as well as a professional, and those lines can be blurred at times. As a nurse I have been able to make a difference in my patient's lives by preparing them to face their cancer treatment, accommodating them while hospitalized, educating them daily and comforting them through their most critical time. Dealing with a cancer diagnosis, its treatment and its aftermath can be daunting for even the most well-adjusted individual with the best support system. I have been blessed to be a part of many patient journeys and I wouldn't trade this for anything else.

~

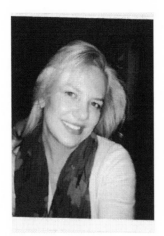

Janet Villalobos, ARNP is a Board Certified Acute Care Nurse Practitioner working in Pain Management at the University of Miami, Sylvester
Comprehensive Cancer Center, where she focuses mainly on cancer pain.
She has worked as a registered nurse with over 15 years of healthcare
experience in different specialty areas including pediatric oncology and
ICU nursing, medical/surgical telemetry, home health, case management
and adult oncology.

21

PALLIATIVE CARE - IT'S NEVER TOO EARLY

MARIANA KHAWAND, M.D. AND KHIN M. ZAW. M.D.

"Palliative Care."

Quite often – and incorrectly – these words are associated with "giving up" in the medical world. When they hear the words, "palliative care," people feel sadness. They become scared and uncomfortable, and in many cases, shut down emotionally, refusing to listening to any further on the subject.

But this is all a big misunderstanding.

The simplest definition and purpose of palliative care? Improving the quality of life for individuals with serious illnesses.

As palliative care physicians, we typically spend a great deal of time explaining its meaning to patients and colleagues, with an emphasis on how it can help anyone coping with a serious or chronic medical condition, regardless of prognosis and whether it's curable.

But before we discuss what palliative care is, it's important to note what palliative care is NOT:

- Palliative care is not just for dying patients;
- Palliative care is not the inevitable outcome when doctors

have determined there's "no hope," or that they "have done everything they can;
- Palliative care is not the same as hospice care;
- Palliative care is not just about administering strong pain medications to sick patients;
- Palliative care is not physician-assisted suicide or euthanasia;
- Palliative care is not only for patients with incurable illnesses or for whom curative treatment has failed.

What is Palliative Care?

Palliative care is the name given for treatment of the discomfort, symptoms, and stress of serious illnesses like cancer, COPD, and heart failure. The palliative care approach takes more than just a patient's disease into consideration; it also addresses his or her spirituality, life goals, family dynamics, functionality, and even financial concerns.

This comprehensive approach to patient care allows palliative care teams to fully understand a person's core values and what is most important to them during their journey through life with a chronic illness. Palliative care teams often help patients and their families digest the influx of medical information coming at them from various specialties and devise a plan of care that is most appropriate for their individual values and goals.

Although palliative care is still a growing field, its role in cancer care has been well-established for many years now. Both cancer and its treatments often lead to undesirable symptoms including:

- Pain
- Fatigue
- Nausea
- Loss of appetite
- Insomnia

Of course, we could add many more to that list.

Sometimes the symptoms a patient experiences are so unpleasant and overwhelming that they interfere with and interrupt treatment plans. One common example is chemotherapy, when side effects like nausea and fatigue simply become too severe for the patient to continue. Palliative care teams help cancer patients cope with the side effects of treatment as well as the impact cancer and cancer treatment impose on their lives in general. Late on in this chapter, we will discuss the many benefits of early palliative care in diseases like cancer.

While many doctors across the varied specialties treat symptoms of serious illness, a palliative care specialist brings special training and expertise in pain management and symptom control for chronic illnesses to his practice. Furthermore, palliative care physicians work in an interdisciplinary team that includes palliative care nurses, psychologists, social workers, and chaplains. This team may also include nutritionists, pharmacists, physical therapists, recreational therapists, and other valuable members who can provide a holistic approach to patients with cancer and other serious illnesses.

Palliative care teams help patients not only with medical management of symptoms and side effects, but also with patient and family stress revolving around sickness, fears about the future, and guidance in choosing treatment options aligned with a patient's overall goals of care. One of a palliative care physician's many roles is to discuss treatment options and help patients navigate through their journey.

You may hear the phrase "quality of life" employed by many in the medical setting. The palliative care team is essentially a task force dedicated to maximizing this very aspect of taking care of YOU: the quality of *your* life as *you* define it.

How Does the Palliative Care Team Provide This Support?

Palliative care physicians most commonly see patients when they are hospitalized. Generally, a palliative care "consultation" is requested by your primary doctor in the hospital. Often, the purpose of this consultation is to serve the purpose of managing difficult symptoms and/or discussing your "goals of care" to help guide you through tough medical decisions.

Unfortunately, palliative care teams are often consulted at the later stage of illness, or when symptoms are too difficult to control with standard management. This is a regrettable byproduct of the common misperception surrounding palliative care: that it is exclusively for the end of someone's life. But let us assure you, it is not.

Palliative care can help countless people with many years yet to live!

In the hospital setting, one of the most commons symptoms addressed by palliative care specialists is pain. Pain management using strong medications called "opioids" requires a specific set of skills for which palliative care specialists receive training. This training includes a thorough understanding of what kinds of pain will respond to what kinds of medication, along with their possible side effects and safe usage.

Palliative care physicians also address and work to alleviate nausea, vomiting, constipation, diarrhea, depression, anxiety, insomnia, fatigue, lack of concentration, problems with walking or performing daily activities, and the emotional and social stress that accompanies being diagnosed with a serious or chronic disease.

Aside from recommending medications for pain and other symptoms in the hospital, palliative care teams are also asked to help when patients and families face difficult decisions about how to proceed with treatment; they also assist in discussions about *advance directives* – the name given to your wishes in the event you're unable to express yourself at the time of medical decision-making. This is accomplished through a careful review of your medical records, consultations with the multiple specialists involved in your care, and most importantly, conversations with *you*.

The members of the palliative care team, including the doctors, will spend a lot of time speaking with you in order to understand and determine what is most important to you. The types of questions posed by palliative care specialists are:

- What do you understand about your illness?
- How do you prefer to hear medical information – are you a "big picture" person, or do you prefer to know all the details?
- What brings you joy in life?
- How has your illness affected your ability to enjoy your life or do what you need to do?
- Who is closest to you? Who would make decisions on your behalf if you were unable?
- What is your faith or belief system?
- Do you consider yourself spiritual or religious?
- What things do you believe in that give meaning to your life?
- How important is your faith or belief system? What influence does it have on how you take care of yourself?
- How have your beliefs influenced your behavior during this illness? What role do they play in regaining your health?
- Are you a part of a spiritual or religious community? Is this of support to you? How? Is there an individual or a group of people you really love, or who are of utmost importance to you?
- As your healthcare provider, how would you like me to address these issues in your healthcare?

Through the process of spending time getting to know you, reviewing your medical history, and discussing your care with all of your specialists, palliative care doctors and team members can help you navigate through decision-making as it pertains to your medical care by discussing options and providing medical opinion. After palliative care consultation, patients tend to have a deeper sense of what's most dear to them over the course of their illness.

In some hospitals, palliative care teams are automatically notified of any patients entering the hospital who have a past or current diagnosis of cancer; advanced heart, lung, or liver disease; or other chronic illnesses. Consequently, someone from the palliative care team will meet with these patients. From there, they can help determine whether or not the patient will benefit from seeing a palliative care specialist outside of the hospital. The team can also help patients define their goals and prioritize them in the context of their illnesses. This "reflex palliative care consultation" is becoming more and more popular as this medical specialty continues to grow.

Thus far, we've only discussed palliative care in the hospital.

Though still an evolving and expanding part of the field, outpatient palliative care practices are beginning to emerge throughout the county, especially at large cancer centers.

Going to an outpatient palliative care practice means that aside from seeing your primary care doctor, oncologist, radiation oncologist, and any other specialists, you'll have additional support for your pain and symptom management. Although it may seem daunting to add yet another specialist to your list of doctors, most people enjoy their visits to palliative care practices, due to the focus on well-being and big-picture type considerations.

These office visits often consist of chronic pain management, discussion and management of other distressing symptoms, and conversations about advance care planning and care goals. During each visit, your palliative care practitioner will work closely with you to ensure you still have good quality of life while undergoing treatment for your cancer – or even for years afterward – in order to address the residual side effects or symptoms of cancer treatment.

Outpatient palliative care practices often network with supportive care services. These include outpatient psychologists, psychiatrists, integrative medicine specialists, and interventional pain specialists.

Integrative medicine specialists are medical doctors who focus on lifestyle and nutrition. Thus, they can offer some alternative options for patients including acupuncture and herbal and plant-based medicine.

Interventional pain specialists treat pain with intricate procedures including pain management pump placement, injections called "nerve blocks," and multiple other procedures to alleviate pain that is not well controlled by medications. Your palliative care specialist will involve these other specialties to give you a comprehensive approach to a good quality of life. Your palliative care physician will also keep in touch with your primary care physician as well as any other specialists involved in your care – from oncologists who provide medical treatment for cancer to surgeons, to radiation oncologists who specialize in the use of radiation for cancer treatment.

Besides focusing on quality of life through management of symptoms, palliative care specialists address who you are as a person – not just your medical history. Many initial visits last well over an hour, both in the hospital and in the office setting.

Why?

Palliative care physicians want to know who you are, what is important to you, and how you cope with adversity. Combined with medical knowledge, this information allows palliative care physicians to guide you through complicated medical decisions.

Finally, your outpatient palliative care team will assist you with "advance care planning." This involves discussion about your preferences in your medical care, should you become unable to communicate. This process works most efficiently when it includes the people closest to you, so they are fully aware of your wishes. Palliative care physicians and other providers can help you put these wishes into writing. As your health status changes, your palliative care doctor will revisit the topic and update your documents as necessary.

An Example of Palliative Care in Action

To paint a fuller picture of what it's like to receive help from a palliative care team, let us tell you the story of Jane – a fictional patient whom we'll use to illustrate what a palliative care team does.

Jane Smith is a 45 year-old woman with breast cancer who is currently at the Saint Elsewhere Cancer Center receiving an infusion of chemotherapy. While at chemotherapy, she experiences nausea and vomiting, then faints. She is then transferred to the hospital for rehydration and observation. During her hospitalization, Jane continues to have very severe nausea and vomiting. She reports to her doctors that she also has a lot of pain and tingling in both of her feet, and that the pain meds she takes at home no longer work for her.

The palliative care team is called upon for help with managing Jane's nausea and vomiting as well as her pain.

Dr. Kay, a palliative care physician, meets with Jane to discuss these undesirable symptoms and side effects. Through this conversation, Dr. Kay also discovers that Kay has been very unhappy lately because her foot pain has been preventing her from participating in her favorite activity – dancing. Jane also confides to Dr. Kay that she's worried about her children, who rely on her for help with homework. She also admits that since her cancer diagnosis, she's been struggling with insomnia, a poor appetite, and a general lack of motivation.

In response, Dr. Kay administers stronger medications for nausea, vomiting, and pain. While Jane is in the hospital, Dr. Kay and her team visit her every day. In three days, Jane improves and is ready to return home.

Before she leaves the hospital however, Dr. Kay and the palliative care team work together to ensure that Jane's concerning issues are being addressed. Together, Dr. Kay and Jane create a list of Jane's most important goals:

- She wants her pain under control so she can resume her dance classes

- She wants to be awake and alert enough to help her kids with their homework
- She wants to stop losing weight
- She wants to maintain her strength
- She wants to continue chemotherapy and live as long as possible so she can be around for her kids
- She wants to feel happier

Dr. Kay, with the help of the palliative care pharmacists, recommends a stronger set of medicines for Jane. The team also suggests a medication to help with concentration and energy on those days when she's feeling tired or requiring more of the pain medications that make her sleepy.

The social worker and nurse then meet with Jane to ensure she's able to get her new prescriptions and that her insurance will cover them.

The team nutritionist talks with Jane about foods that are more palatable to her, offering recommendations on which ones will help her maintain her weight and reduce nausea.

The psychologist speaks with Jane about her issues with moodiness and recommends an outpatient therapist who can continue to guide her through this very difficult period of her life. At this time, Jane is not interested in taking depression or anxiety medications.

On the first day they met, Dr. Kay asked Jane about her spirituality. Jane shared that she'd been raised Catholic and that previously, her faith had been source of comfort. However, now she's not so sure if her religion can help her. She'd agreed to meet with the team's chaplain, who helped her seek silent meditation and create a space to reconnect with her spirituality.

Finally, the team communicated with Jane's oncologist and primary doctor to apprise them of the plan moving forward, including her new medications. Dr. Kay advises Jane to follow up at her palliative care office on a monthly basis to monitor her pain management and other symptoms.

During her one-month follow-up, Jane reports she's feeling better and tolerating the chemotherapy much better, thanks to her new nausea medications. Although she still has pain in her feet, it is somewhat improved. While it's not possible for her to tolerate dance classes yet, she feels she's moving closer to that goal.

She continues to see Dr. Kay at the office to help her with her symptoms. At one point Dr. Kaye refers Jane to the integrative medicine doctor, who helps Jane with her sleeping habits and offers acupuncture for her anxiety.

Over the course of her visits, Jane talks with Dr. Kay about her wishes in the event she should become too sick to make medical decisions on her own. She designates her husband as her "surrogate decision maker" and completes advance directive paperwork – so that if does become sick in the future her family will have some guidance in how to proceed.

In the beginning, these conversations made Jane and her husband uncomfortable, but now they are grateful to have completed this step in planning their future. Doing so has given Jane a feeling of control over her cancer. Additionally, this will be extremely helpful in guiding Jane's husband and family should she ever become severely ill. Now they have a deeper understanding about her preferences, so that instead of feeling forced to make tough decisions without any guidance, they'll have a clearers sense of what to do.

Jane's cancer responds very well to chemotherapy and she continues to follow up with Dr. Kay to manage her foot pain.

Jane's story is just one simplified example of how a palliative care team can help a patient through many of the challenges of sickness, even in non-life-threatening situations. Thanks to Jane's time spent with Dr. Kay and her team in the hospital and at the office, she now has an improved quality of life and a deeper understanding of her health.

When Should I Ask About Palliative Care?

The truth is, it's never too early to involve a palliative care team once a patient has been diagnosed with a serious illness. The medical condition does *not* have to be incurable or life-limiting.

Palliative care services are often underutilized because many patients – and even doctors – unfortunately equate "palliative care" with "end-of-life care." We often overhear our well-meaning colleagues in the medical field stating, "there is nothing else we can do; let's just switch to palliative care."

We urge our colleagues and patients to see it in a different light. Palliative care should be provided ALONGSIDE all other care – not as an alternative or last resort. The medical team does not have to "switch" to palliative care; they can add palliative care to the total care of a patient to improve the patient's quality of life.

So, if you are diagnosed with cancer or any other chronic or serious illness, and you have pain or other symptoms, palliative care can be of service. If you're faced with a difficult medical decision and need guidance, palliative can help. If you're having difficulty coping with the impact of a serious illness, palliative care is there for you.

Surely not everyone needs every aspect of palliative care, but everyone can benefit from reflecting upon what's important to them as a person, not just a patient. Conversations with palliative care teams are almost always guaranteed to help patients – whether by gaining a better understanding of their illness, reflecting more deeply upon the goals of care, or by alleviating distressing symptoms.

The most important thing to remember is that the core purpose of palliative care as a specialty is to improve quality of life in the setting of the illness. We do this through pain and symptom management, addressing you as a whole person, gaining a fuller understanding of your core values and goals, and guiding you in your journey through life with a serious illness. This holistic approach to patient care forms the very foundation of palliative care.

A Brief Overview of Hospice Care – Palliative Care at the End of Life

Oftentimes, palliative care is confused with hospice care – the name for palliative care given at the end of life. Hospice care always includes palliative care, but palliative care does not always include hospice care.

Hospice is a set of services and benefits offered to patients at the end of life. It can be delivered at home, at a nursing home or assisted living facility, or in an inpatient hospice unit in a hospital or other facility. In-hospital hospice care is usually reserved for patients who need specialized care such as intravenous (IV) medications, or for patients who have symptoms difficult to manage at home.

Once enrolled in hospice, a hospice organization provides many services to maximize patients' quality of life. Home oxygen tanks, a hospital bed for the home, and other medical equipment are all provided by the hospice benefit. Patients receive daily visits from home attendants to help with bathing (if necessary) and other daily needs. A nurse comes to visit the patient at home at least once a week – sometimes more often – to check vital signs, arrange medications, and perform other medical tasks such as wound care. A hospice physician will come and visit once a month or more frequently as needed, to take care of prescriptions and examine the patient.

When patients become ill or have uncontrolled symptoms, the hospice nurse will notify the hospice organization and that the patient can be put on "continuous care." This means there will be health aides at the house 24 hours a day, a nurse will visit daily, and the doctors will visit up to once a day if needed. It's basically like having hospital-level care and supervision without the patient ever having to leave the comfort of home.

Home hospice allows patients to avoid admittance to the hospital and maximize comfort toward the end of life. Many people who enroll in hospice actually live longer than expected! There are many explanations for this, including the fact that being at home and experiencing such focused care prevents more setbacks and returns to the hospital.

If however, the patient requires IV medications, special procedures, or any service or intervention that cannot be delivered at home, he or she can go to an inpatient hospice unit. These units can be located inside a hospital or in a separate building. Inpatient hospice units are equipped with nurse and staff trained to care for hospice patients. A hospice/palliative care physician will see the patient daily while they are in the inpatient hospice unit receiving treatments.

When patients do reach the end of life, many prefer to pass away at home, while others prefer to be under the care of doctors and nurses in a hospice unit. Hospice teams honor patients' wishes and provide support for patients and their families during these difficult times. Bereavement services, more commonly known as grief counseling services, are often included in the hospice benefit after a loved one has passed away.

In addition, hospice teams have social workers, psychologists, chaplains, and other trained specialists who help patients and families cope with the dying process. These team members are available both in the home hospice setting (including nursing homes and assisted living facilities) as well as in the inpatient hospice units.

The focus in hospice is patient comfort. Generally, at this stage of a patient's illness there are no attempts at curing the disease because no curative options exist; because the patient cannot tolerate the curative treatments; or because the patient and family decline curative treatments, due to their personal wishes and in order to maintain quality of life.

It's important to realize however, that hospice does not mean "do not treat." Routinely, patients under the hospice benefit are still given antibiotics for infections, blood transfusions for symptoms of low blood counts, and other treatments for other illnesses that arise. Patients on hospice continue their routine medications for their other medical conditions. For example, in the case of someone receiving the hospice benefit because of metastatic lung cancer, that person continues their routine diabetes, blood pressure, and cholesterol medications.

Another important misconception about hospice that must be addressed is the belief that hospice doctors "just give you medicine to help you die faster." This could not be further from the truth!

Hospice teams focus on comfort, and in the final days of life morphine is a great tool employed to treat pain and shortness of breath. The doses of morphine used are safe and effective for treating symptoms, but not high enough to cause death.

Any physician or palliative care team can discuss hospice and whether or not it is appropriate for you or someone you love.

The hospice approach to patients is 100% palliative care – patient-centered, comfort-oriented care that takes into consideration the physical, emotional, social, and spiritual aspects of a person's life.

While hospice care is only appropriate in specific situations, palliative care is appropriate for any age, for any diagnosis, at any stage of a serious illness. It's provided together with curative and life-prolonging treatments.

RESOURCES FOR HOSPICE AND PALLIATIVE CARE

1. Information on advance directives: www.caringinfo.org
2. National Hospice and Palliative Care Organization: www.nhpco.org
3. Palliative Care Provider Resource: www.getpalliativecare.org
4. National Institutes of Health Resources for Patients and Providers on Symptom Management and Other Issues in Palliative Care: www.nlm.nih.gov/medlineplus/palliativecare.html

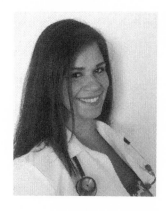

Dr. Mariana Khawand-Azoulai was born in Beirut Lebanon. Shortly thereafter, her parents moved to Miami Florida, where she spent her entire youth. She minored in mathematics and earned a bachelor's degree in Microbiology and Immunology, and a B.A. in Chemistry from the University of Miami. Dr. Khawand-Azoulai also holds a Master's in Physiology from Georgetown University, which she followed up with four years of medical school at the University of Florida in Gainesville. After completing her residency in Family Medicine at Columbia/New York Presbyterian Hospital, she's now training in a one-year fellowship in Hospice and Palliative Medicine at the University of Miami/Jackson Hospital healthcare system. She currently resides in Miami with her husband Yoni, an Emergency Medicine Physician at the University of Miami Hospital, and their two daughters.

Contact Dr. Mariana Khawand-Azoulai at Dr.Khawand@gmail.com.

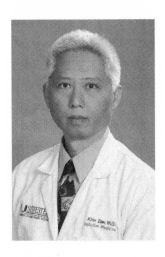

Dr. Khin Maung Zaw was born in Moulmein, Burma (Myanmar). He received his medical degree from Institute of Medicine (2), Rangoon, Burma and practiced general medicine in rural and urban settings before immigrating to the United States in 1992. He completed his internal medicine residency at St. Barnabas Hospital in Bronx, New York before starting a successful VA career including Fargo VA and Buffalo VA. He completed his VA Interprofessional Palliative Care Fellowship at Palo Alto VAMC in 2004 and the Geriatric Medicine Fellowship at Montefiore Medical Center, Bronx, New York in 2005. He is boarded in Internal Medicine, Geriatric Medicine, and Hospice and Palliative Medicine. During his career as palliative care physician at the Miami VA from 2005 to 2012, he founded a comprehensive palliative care program with a grant from the VA Central Office. As a full-time faculty member at the University of Miami, Dr. Zaw is responsible for the growth of the palliative care program, including the establishment of the outpatient palliative care clinic at Sylvester Comprehensive Cancer Center. He is the founding director of the Hospice and Palliative Medicine Fellowship program; ACGME accredited in 2014. He currently resides in Miami Florida with his family.

Contact Dr. Khin Maung Zaw at kzaw@med.miami.edu.

335

22

BECOMING A FEARLESS CAREGIVER

GARY BARG

Becoming a Fearless Caregiver

When the phone rang in her South Florida home one summer after-noon, Monica knew all too well about the life changes that some phone calls can bring. A few years earlier, shortly after her husband Bob's retirement, they received a call from the family doctor, advising Bob to report immediately to the local hospital, only days after a routine physical examination. Bob had been diagnosed with Multiple Myeloma and passed away within a year. This time the phone call came from Monica's father's doctor, the diagnosis was in and Joe, her dad, was living with Alzheimer's disease. The long road of family caregiving began anew.

In the case of her father, Monica was, like so many other senior caregivers so few years ago, faced with the challenges of caregiving without the benefit of any long-term care insurance. Within the next five years, all of Joe's savings, accumulated over sixty years of a productive work life were depleted and the financial burden on Monica and her family was becoming staggering, as they not only cared for Joe but also his wife, Helen. Between them, Joe and Helen were dealing with cancer, Alzheimer's strokes and diabetes. How do I know so much about this family? Because Monica is my mother.

Before you think that my family's situation is so unique, consider the fact that, at present, there are over 65 million other family caregivers in the United States. These caregivers are responsible for the lives and well being of their loved ones who need care. They are also commonly referred to as the "Sandwich Generation" since they find themselves sandwiched between responsibilities to parents as well as to children, grandchildren and spouses. Recently the recognition of multi-generational caregiving has even been extended to include the phrase "Club Sandwich Generation" referring to the fact that in some families, caregiving can include members of more than three generations.

When I returned home to South Florida during the summer of 1994 to help my mom as she cared for Joe and Helen, I thought the trip home would last for two weeks, at the most. I planned to be there long enough to help mom make some decisions concerning my grandparents, look over some paperwork, offer support and be back on my way to Atlanta, were I was living and working as a video producer, getting ready to produce work for the upcoming 1996 Olympics. Yet, before I unpacked my suitcase on the first day of my visit home, things were already in full swing. We received a call from the facility where Gramp was living. He had been living in an assisted living facility since his afore-mentioned Alzheimer's diagnoses and recently, his behavior had changed to the point where more oversight was necessary, and the facility was insistent that we move him immediately. My grandmother had taken a fall, which combined with her intense depression and strokes, made the multiple doctor visits necessary for her care a physical challenge for Mom.

The third night I was back in town, I accompanied Mom on a supermarket shopping trip for my grandmother and her home care aide, who had given Mom a grocery list to follow. Mom told me that she had just been to the store recently and couldn't understand how they could have gone through so much food. I was overwhelmed by the number of staples these two women seemingly needed. A five-pound bag of sugar, a large bag of rice, ten pounds of chuck steak, etc, all items which mom had purchased not two weeks ago. I suggested that we stop by the apartment unannounced that very evening rather than wait until the next morning as the aide had suggested. At first, when we walked into the apartment, I thought I had opened the wrong door. There were at least five adults and a dozen kids running around, all burners were cooking food and my grandmother was left alone in her bedroom. I ushered the aide and her extended family out of the apartment and we stayed with my grandmother until a suitable replacement was found. Our first mistake as novice care-givers was not doing a thorough background check on the aide, having hired her on the suggestion of a friend of a friend of the fami-ly's. Although, I have become an advocate of using professional services such as an agency or a registry, good support can be found from independent service providers, if you learn how to do your homework regardless of which option you use to find support.

The second mistake was sticking to a visiting schedule suggested by the home care aide. No matter how comfortable you are with the in-home service provider, you should either stop by on an irregular schedule or if that is not possible due to long distance caregiving, ask a local friend or relative to keep an eye on your loved one or utilize the services of a local care manager.

At the end of my two-week visit, as mom and I sat on the couch in her house exhausted from the constant challenges presented by caring for our family members, I turned to her and said, "You know, I'm glad that I was able to visit during these particular two weeks due to all that went on." She looked at me blankly and asked, "What are you talking about?" It dawned on me that while I thought these two weeks represented an unusual roller-coaster ride of healthcare, finan-cial and mental challenges; to Mom it was just another few weeks in her life as a caregiver. I returned to Atlanta long enough to gather my belongings and move back home for the duration. I had become what I like to call a caregiver's caregiver. I was going to do whatever was necessary to support mom as she helped to make our relatives lives as comfortable and as safe as possible. A few months later, after visiting my grandmother during one of her many hospital stays, I had lunch in a restaurant on Miami Beach. In front of me on the restaurant table, was spread the mountains of paperwork I had to sort through as a caregiver. These included flyers from the Alzheimer's Association, brochures from a variety of Assisted Living Facilities and a huge pile of insurance papers. It occurred to me that there must be a better way to organize this information for caregivers and that they deserved all the help that could be found. Although my background was in video and film, it seemed that a magazine was a better media to create to more quickly distribute to caregivers in need. But first, I would have to do some research; it was utterly impossible that there wouldn't already be such a publication out there, Bankers had magazines, Floor manufacturers had magazines; there certainly must have already been a magazine available for family caregivers. Over the next few weeks, I looked in every library and bookstore in the area (this was before Internet Search Engines) and could find nothing.

So, we decided that if such a publication were indeed needed, we would have to create it ourselves. I went to the local mall and bought a computer, printer, paper and ink and kept my fingers crossed that I could put it all together. I will never forget the look on my mom's face as I lugged all this equipment into an available bedroom in her home, where we were to set up our first office for Today's Caregiver magazine.

Mom immediately stepped up to the plate and from the first issue of the magazine, would write insightful, honest and supportive articles about topics that she knew would be of importance to her fellow caregivers. Frankly, she would be writing about issues that she was dealing with herself. They included such topics as the challenges faced getting other family members to help, the death of her brother, her bouts with depression and dealing with medical professionals.

The next 23 years flew by quickly. During this time, in my conversations with many thousands of family caregivers, one thing has become crystal clear, family caregivers must not remain the silent chaperone sitting in the corner of the examining room as our loved one is attended to by his or her doctor. We have a voice that can be heard and respected by the members of our loved one's care team. In fact, we must learn to become leading members of the team. Just as the other members have jobs to do, so do you. Yours is to put a human face to your loved one; many times, these care professionals are not seeing your loved one as you know them to be. You need to help remind them of who your loved one is, was and has been.

On becoming a Fearless Caregiver

I watched out of the corner of my eye as a family caregiver attendee strode across the large banquet hall at one of our Fearless Caregiver conferences. She was on a determined mission to reach her destination and would not be deterred. And I was afraid that destination was me. This event was held in our own hometown of Fort Lauderdale where the first event was also held in 1998. To me, the linchpin of the events is always the Question and Answer session which usually occur early in the day's agenda. This is the time where the audience members can get to ask any question they wish of a panel of local and national care experts. These panels usually include a social worker, local caregiver resource expert, nurse, and on occasion, both a doctor and a lawyer. More likely than not the panelists are able to answer any question thrust upon them. I would run around the audience with a wireless microphone doing my best to elicit the questions from the caregivers in the audience. Frankly, it is most fun for me during these sessions when a question would arise that the panel of experts could not answer. I like to call this the "Stump the Panel" moment. Not in any way to embarrass our experts, but because I know for a fact that the other group of caregiving experts in the room will be up to the task and answer with many appropriate and innovate responses. The experts I refer to of course are always our roomful of family caregivers. And that is the main reason for the exercise of answering audience questions in the first place, to illustrate to caregivers that knowledge was not a one-way street, they (or other caregivers like them) already had more answers than they could have imagined before the questions ever started flowing in the session. After the caregiver striding across the room finally reached me, she whispered in my ear as I pointed the microphone at another caregiver about to ask a question of our caregiving panel. What she whispered was this: "I have a question that I think is too stupid to ask in public and so I would like you to ask it for me". Gee thanks. I quickly pointed the microphone in her direction and announced to the assemblage," This lady has a question to ask of us." There was one reason for my response and it had nothing to do with cruelty.

In fact, one other thing I do know is that whatever question this caregiver standing before me would ask, it would be poignant, appropriate and the furthest thing from stupid. Unfortunately, the specific question is lost in the haze of time, but I will always remember what happened next. The lawyer who was serving on the Question and Answer panel of experts, upon hearing the question, slammed the table and said; "I've been waiting all morning for someone to ask that very question." The caregiver glided back to her seat on a cushion of air. My confidence in my actions was easy to explain; in the many years that we have been hosting the Fearless Caregiver conferences and in the thousands of emails I have received from family caregivers since launching Today's Caregiver magazine and caregiver.com, I have never once received a silly or inappropriate question from a family caregiver. Never. This brings us to the first rule of Fearless Caregiving: Any question you have as a family caregiver is important and deserves to be answered quickly, concisely and with the respect you deserve as a member of your loved one's care team.

The truth is that the role we caregivers play in the care of our loved ones can not easily be overstated. On average, a caregiver will be responsible for the directed expenditures of over $40,000 a year caring for their loved one (make it $47,000 for Alzheimer's care), and out of pocket - almost ten percent of his or her annual salary -- they will lose over $600,000 in opportunities and promotions during the lifetime of their career and over 63% of caregivers will consider depression to be their most commonly felt emotion. And according to a recent Stanford University study, nearly 30% of us will die before our loved ones do.

Then why do we do it? The answer is simple...we can't not do it. It is because our loved ones need us. Because we never even asked ourselves if there was any other way. Because it's who we are. So, now what? How do we go from being partner and spouse or dedicated daughter or son to be a dietitian, therapist, insurance specialist, immediate medical expert, chauffer, psychologist, pharmacist and incontinence specialist? And keep our relationship with our loved ones, families, friends and neighbors. Not to mention our jobs, which a third of us end up losing.

I firmly believe the way that that we achieve our goals as caregivers is by taking on a new job role. That is one I call being a Fearless Caregiver. A Fearless Caregiver is a caregiver who understands that they have a job to do as a full member of their loved one's care team. You all have jobs to do and yours is to learn all you can about your loved one's situation and act as their advocate.

You are there not only to represent your loved one but also to put a human face to them. This is a crucial role, no matter how much they care, your doctor sees at least 25 patients a day, your case manager and therapist have a larger case load than ever, and other members of a hospital or care facilities team probably has never even laid eyes on your loved one. A family caregiver can be heard in today's healthcare system and we can be listened to. Over the years, we have found three significant common traits among the caregivers who are being heard. The first is that they must believe that they can make a difference. Second, they see their role in their loved one's care as being just as important as any of the professional caregivers. And third, they ask questions. They ask lots of questions. They research and do not easily take "no" for an answer. They become Fearless Caregivers.

A Fearless Caregiver is one who asks questions of their doctor and does not rest until they receive clear and concise answers. A Fearless Caregiver knows their rights concerning their loved one's insurance plan and can exercise those rights. A Fearless Caregiver is one who knows how to find the latest treatment options and present qualified research to the members of her loved one's care team. A Fearless Caregiver IS a member of their loved one's care team.

Yet, do you know what the very first step to such care is? – it is caring for yourself. I can hear you saying as you read these words "who has time to care for me, I spend all my time caring for him (or her)?" My answer to that is, who will care for you AND your loved one when you take ill due to exhaustion or simply not caring for yourself. See, Job One for any caregiver is to make sure that we are taken care of, too.

Recently at another Fearless Caregiver conference, that fact came alive for me as well as all caregivers in attendance. The event was held in Palm Beach County, Florida and the weather were as close to a tropical storm as it could be without the news stations going into full soap opera interruption mode. I had broken three of my cardinal rules about hosting these events and they are: stay north in the warm months, south in the cold months, and avoid Florida during the hurricane season. Thankfully, there was a lull in the weather during the time that people normally arrive for the events and we had a packed house of hundreds of caregivers. Just after the applause died down after our luncheon speaker's session ended, I took the stage and before I was able to utter a word, heard someone cry from the audience" Is there a doctor in the house?" Not something you want to hear at any event, let alone one you are hosting. I stopped the proceedings and went to the center of the room to find a nicely dressed grey haired lady slumped over in her chair. There were no doctors in the house but plenty of nurses and as I reached the table, two nurses were already assessing the situation. They lady mentioned that she felt like she was going to pass out. We called 911 and they were there within minutes. She was at the event was with her husband, a gentleman sitting calmly next to her who was living with Alzheimer's disease, and she was, of course, most concerned about his care.

The paramedics suggested that she go to the hospital with them and she refused, but they insisted, stating that she would probably just relapse once she got home. They had a tough time getting any information from her and finally she told them that she had a son who lived in town. He was contacted and advised to meet his parents at the hospital. As she left, she told one of my associates that she stays up worrying abut her husband all night and that she never takes care of herself.

Some of her friends coaxed her to attend the event knowing that she needed help; but was not willing to accept any and hoped that she could learn something about the importance of taking care of herself as a caregiver while at the conference. I think we all did.

The Fearless Caregiver conference series began in 1998 when we wanted to bring a group of family and professional caregivers, as well as local and national advocates together for the day. The late television actor Robert Urich was the keynote speaker for that first event, having recently shared his cancer diagnosis and remission on national television. Two things were evident throughout the day, the first thing was that caregivers loved to share with one another, and the advice they had to share was as effective and appropriate as they could ever have been found from any degreed professional. And many times, much more so. The reason for this is simple: the family caregiver is the person caring for their loved one around the clock and intuitively creating solutions for the challenges that they faced daily. The other thing that was evident was that caregivers with loved ones with differing diagnoses and caregiving situations could learn from one another's experiences.

As illustration, I recall a luncheon table during that first conference with four caregivers sitting around it. Their main care concern was (respectively) Breast Cancer, Parkinson's, and Alzheimer's disease. As I listened in on them, they were reveling in the fact that each of them brought different but powerful experiences to the table. The caregiver whose primary care concern was breast cancer talked about managing his loved one's medication regime, the Alzheimer's caregiver was sharing her challenges with the long-term care facility in which she had just placed her loved one and the Parkinson's caregiver was talking of solutions he had come up with regards to his loved ones increasing limited mobility. The areas of interest and the skill sets these caregivers brought to that luncheon table were both unique and of specific value to their fellow luncheon companions.

That luncheon group brought to life our concerns about the challenge faced by isolating or "siloing" caregivers based upon their main healthcare issues. For the longest time, caregivers were segmented by the types of disease or illness that their loved one was dealing with. Conferences, publications and even support groups were defined by the disease and not the individual. This fact had come to life for me as I was asked to speak at a wide variety of healthcare conferences: Cancer, Spinal cord, Alzheimer's, Parkinson's or even Scleroderma. Certainly, the medical issues were unique to the diagnoses, but after a while the concerns and the stories of the caregivers I had met at these various events could not have been more similar. They were worried about the best care for their loved ones, had financial concerns, too much stress and too little actionable and appropriate information. Soon, I became somewhat of a healthcare "Johnny Appleseed" spreading the ideas and advice I received from these diverse groups with the next groups I met, regardless of the disease or illness with which their loved ones were dealing. For another event, we were at the Union League Center in downtown Philadelphia and our keynote speaker was the remarkable Della Reese.

Late in the day, a caregiver who had sat silently for most of the day raised her hand to speak. She told us that her mother was in the hospital getting prepped for surgery, but she knew that being with us was too important for her wellbeing to miss. She went on to say that she was the sole informal caregiver for six of her senior neighbors and that she had two heart attacks in the past two years as well as out of control blood pressure. As I asked her to stand and hugged her, the audience took turns giving her advice on caring for herself until a caregiver from across the room stood up and said, "I live in your neighborhood and from now on, you're not alone." Tears flowed from every eye in the room. At the next year's event, these two caregivers and fast friends were sitting next to each other and told the spellbound room of their accomplishments in their respective neighborhood over the past twelve months.

By example the caregivers in the stories above prove that we caregivers must certainly learn all we can about the disease or illness that our loved ones are battling, in this case, knowledge truly is power --- but we must also learn all we can about our role as a caregiver – A Fearless Caregiver.

The first act of any Fearless Caregiver is to assess your resources. Is there a sister, brother, neighbor or professional service that can stand in for you a few hours a week or maybe a weekend every few months? Do you know what community services are available to anyone in your situation? Do you even know where to start looking? As one of the members of our internet support group at caregiver.com put it, "The cemetery is filled with irreplaceable people." Who takes over when the irreplaceable caregiver is gone? If you don't believe you have the right to take care of your own needs, you may need a caregiver yourself.

Unfortunately, too many caregivers die from a combination of stress, depression and ill health. Or, we become unable to care for ourselves, let alone our loved one, leaving a larger question of the healthcare system unanswered; "Who will care for both the caregiver and loved one, when the caregiver becomes ill?"

The good news is that there is a path to ensuring your loved one receives the best care possible without sacrificing your own health. And that is to fearlessly and lovingly adhere to the principle that that caring for yourself is Job One.

~

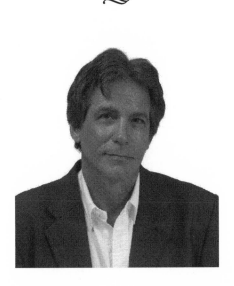

Gary Edward Barg is a noted speaker, writer and publisher on caregiving issues since 1995, Gary Barg is Founder and Editor-In-Chief of *Today's Caregiver*, the first national magazine for caregivers, and the original online caregiver community, www.caregiver.com. *Today's Caregiver* magazine and www.caregiver.com combine information, advice and reader's stories with interviews of celebrity caregivers such as Leeza Gibbons, Rob Lowe, Dana Reeve, Barbara Eden, and Debbie Reynolds, among others. Gary created *The Fearless Caregiver Conferences*, hosted across the country, which bring caregivers together to share their knowledge, experience, and wisdom. His book, *The Fearless Caregiver*, is filled with practical advice, poetry, and inspirational stories. His new book, *Caregiving Ties that Bind* include many of the over 150 celebrity caregiver cover interviews he has conducted since 1995.

His awards include the *Mature Media Award* for writing, *International Television Association Golden Reel Award* and the *Southern Gerontological Society Media Award*.

Gary serves as a member of the Board of Trustees, *National Adult Day Services Association* and a Member of the Board, *American Association for Caregiver Education*.

His interviews include: *The Today Show, Bloomberg Radio Network, Time Magazine, The Wall Street Journal, USA Today, Miami Herald, NPR Diane Rehm Show, Los Angeles Business Journal,* and *Parade Magazine.*

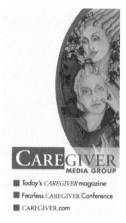

CAREGIVER
MEDIA GROUP

▓ Today's *CAREGIVER* magazine
▓ Fearless CAREGIVER Conference
▓ CAREGIVER.com

23

MALE BREAST CANCER

SAM RIVERA

My name is Samuel Rivera, Sam for short, or Sammy as my family calls me. I was born on January 10, 1954 in Santurce, Puerto Rico, the youngest of five children and the only son. My father always told my mother that he would not stop trying until my mother gave him a boy. It was a man thing, my father wanted a boy to carry on the family's last name, Rivera. I was born a healthy, nine-pound baby; however, my mother had to be hospitalized because she developed tuberculosis. Due to my mother's illness, and while she recovered, my father sent my siblings and me to live with different family members. However, every Sunday, he made sure we spent family time together. Family was an important part of our lives.

At the age of five, my youngest sister, Aury, developed heart problems. My parents were advised to move to New York, so she could be seen by a specialist. When she was six, we came to the United States and settled in the Bronx, New York City. We were very poor, and my parents struggled to make sure we had a place to live and food on the table. My father worked as a machinist and my mother a seamstress. The year we moved to New York, I was clowning around in the kitchen, walking on my hands, and accidentally hit a boiling pot of water, which spilled all over my back. I had to be rushed to Fordham Hospital. That same month, my sister was taken to the same hospital for a heart condition. She was deaf-mute, but we communicated with her through sign language. Tragically, she did not make it. Her passing was a sad time for all of us. As you can probably see by now, life was not easy for our family, but there was one thing that we believed: God did not give us more than we could handle.

Growing up in the Bronx was tough. I had to learn to speak English and adjust to a new way of life, which was difficult and challenging. In the 70's it was even harder, thanks to the presence of gangs. Just going to school was scary. After high school graduation, I decided to join one of the biggest gangs in the world: The United States Army. I enlisted with a friend of mine from Brooklyn named Frankie Silos. We did basic training and AIT (Advanced Individual Training) to become infantrymen. We wanted to go to Vietnam and fight for our country. After basic training at Fort Benning, Georgia, with the 197 Infantry Brigade, I received orders to go overseas.

On a routine examination, the doctor noticed a bloody discharge from my left nipple. I tried to explain that it was because I was working out and developing muscle mass. After further testing, in September 1971, I was shocked to learn I had breast cancer. In denial and embarrassed to have what I considered a "women's disease", I argued with the doctor. I thought it was impossible to develop something only women could get. I was only 18 years old. So, I concocted an elaborate story about being stabbed to share with people, including my buddies. Of course, I refused to discuss my need for surgery with anyone.

Still in denial, I told myself I was a soldier and a man – and men should not be dealing with this disease. Because of my breast cancer diagnosis, I qualified for a medical discharge from the Army. But I refused. I wanted to be a soldier and serve my country to the best of my ability. On November 12, 1973, I was honorably discharged from the military. Since it was too embarrassing, I never told anyone what happened to me. Anytime I went to the beach or anywhere I had to remove my tee shirt, I would find a way to cover the scar. To this day, I. still cover it.

Several members of my family have also had breast cancer, including my grandfather, who died at 110 years old, an aunt, and a niece. I learned that breast cancer does not discriminate. My first wife, now deceased, had metastasized Stage IV breast cancer, which spread to her brain. She taught me not to be afraid to discuss my bout with breast cancer and to help other men identify with their disease. I will always remember her telling me that beauty comes from the inside, not the outside. Another member of my family that was touched by cancer was my daughter, Jasmine, who was only 14 at the time. Her cervical cancer was treated with a freezing procedure to kill the cancer cells, instead of a hysterectomy. Thank God this procedure worked, making it possible for her to have children. I always thank God for helping me through my struggles.

I am now retired from Memorial Regional Hospital, where I worked as an Environmental Services Supervisor, and then a Facilities Management Senior Technician. I received the Presidential Service Award for my work with the Hollywood Fire Rescue Emergency Response Team. Now happily married to Carmen, I am also the father to four grown children: Brenda, Jasmine, Sammy and Samantha, and the proud grandfather of 11 grandchildren. I enjoy remodeling houses, helping others, and playing with my dogs and cats. With God's blessing, I intend to live life to the fullest, always putting Him first.

As a survivor of breast cancer, I advise men to be proactive in their own care. If they suspect anything is wrong or something does not feel right, to see a doctor. Also, being positive and never giving up helps deal with any adverse outcomes. The doctor that was instrumental in my late wife's care was Dr. Carmen Calfa, an oncologist. She gave me hope, when I had no hope, and taught me how to deal with the situation of having had breast cancer, an uncommon occurrence among men. Through Dr. Calfa and her staff, I learned much about the services that are available to those who have had cancer in the past or are currently dealing with it, and who to speak to about them.

This year, I became an advocate for more awareness of breast cancer among men, and participated in the Breast Cancer Institute Day of Caring. I was a male model, along with some beautiful ladies and the theme was "Charlie's Angels". As you might have guessed, I was "Charlie" and the ladies were my "angels." I also found a group out of Kansas City, called the *Male Breast Cancer Coalition*, formed by a young man named Bret Miller. Like me, Bret found out he had breast cancer at the age of 17, but because he was a male, he was overlooked for several years. Thankfully, he is doing well.

Bret's group is helping me, and other men like me to discover more information about the disease, including how to avoid feeling shameful about telling others their breast cancer story. I am also a member of the group, *Cancer Grad Community Quad*. To further my breast cancer awareness efforts, I participate in the *Strive for Breast Cancer* walk in Fort Lauderdale. This year I plan to set it up and invite male breast cancer patients and survivors to walk alongside me and their family and friends. I have found a lot of support in the two groups I have joined and participating in different male breast cancer awareness initiatives has also helped me in understanding how men are susceptible to getting the disease, as much as women are. I highly recommend that other men who have had or have breast cancer to also join support groups of this nature; it is reassuring to know that men are not alone in their fight against breast cancer.

Sam Rivera is retired from Memorial Regional Hospital, where he received the Presidential Service Award for his work with Hollywood Fire Rescue Emergency Response Team. Now married to Carmen, he is the father of four adult children: Brenda, Jasmine, Sammy, and Samantha. He enjoys remodeling houses, helping others, and playing with his dogs and cats. Sam intends to live life to the fullest, always putting God first.

24

HEROINES HARMONIZE TO HEAL: I FOUND MY LUMP AND THEN MY VOICE

MARILYN VAN HOUTIN R.N., M.S., C.C.M.

I found the lump while showering.

It was high on my chest wall, firm and pushing through the skin in an unmistakable way. I thought this had something to do with the push-ups I had done in the pool that week. My conscious thought process would not allow me to "go there" with thoughts that this lump could be cancerous. It was not technically in my breast, so that guided me in my positive thought process that it was nothing to do with breast cancer & would just "go away." Within days, it appeared to grow. Now I was getting concerned and called my PCP for an appointment the following week.

My doctor ordered a mammogram and listed the diagnosis as "breast mass." Now I was scared. Eight months earlier, I had a mammogram, which was normal. The report read that it was "off the field," meaning the mammogram didn't go high enough. In previous mammograms there was no ultrasound done. Today, an ultrasound is a given thanks to actress Joan Lunden (a fellow breast cancer survivor) who spoke up about dense breast tissue & the importance of ultrasound in conjunction with mammograms.

After seeing my primary care physician, I was off for a biopsy. The music *Onward Christian Soldiers* was playing in the outpatient center during the biopsy, surprising and soothing me: I remembered every word of that song from church!

Now the situation I was facing was coming into focus and I was officially on the breast cancer roller coaster. After waiting one week, I called my PCP office and begged not to have to wait a second weekend. I was busy at work during the week and I didn't think much about it, but over the weekends when I didn't have as many activities, I worried about the results a lot. I begged the doctor's secretary to have the doctor call me, and then fax over the results.

The call never came, but the fax did. I received my diagnosis OVER THE FAX MACHINE! The report read "invasive ductal carcinoma, high grade, triple negative, comedo necrosis, negative for estrogen, negative for progesterone, negative for HER2." I read the results out loud to my office assistant. When she asked what it all meant I admitted reluctantly, "I have breast cancer." Reading the report over and over, I had no idea what "triple negative" meant. I remember thinking of the term "negative" as being something positive, as it often is in medicine. My personal defense mechanisms had prevented me from believing it could possibly BE breast cancer. No one in my family (to my knowledge at that time) had ever had it, nor did anyone I knew.

I was totally blindsided. I'd refrained from researching it much during those two weeks of waiting, but that all changed the second I read the biopsy report from the fax machine. I stayed up researching on the internet until 2 a.m. that night, and many more nights to follow. In the beginning, out of fear, I did exactly what the doctor said to do, without asking any questions. During my first appointment with the oncologist at Mount Sinai, I remember him saying, "you gave me a very difficult spot to operate on."

Time moved swiftly after my quadrantectomy (partial or segmental mastectomy) – removal of approximately a quarter of the breast tissue, a wide excision of the overlying skin, and of the underlying connective tissue. There seemed to be an urgency to begin the dose-dense chemo, so immediately I became a triple negative breast cancer (TNBC) expert of sorts. It was a brand-new phenotype; it is NOT driven by the hormones estrogen or progesterone or by the overexpression of the protein HER2. Unlike all other types of breast cancer, which can be treated with medications to decease the odds of recurrence, there are no targeted therapies for TNBC.

In fact, some of the doctors knew very little about TNBC characteristics. It is extremely aggressive, tends to re-occur quickly, metastasizes frequently, is often locally advanced (usually in the lymph nodes when diagnosed), and in many cases, effectively treated with chemo. As a Registered Nurse (RN) I always felt "knowledge is power," so I decided to become a knowledgeable warrior. I Googled every article written on TNBC and shared the information with my providers. Via PubMed online, I signed up for every new article on the subject. I wrote to the doctors and research authors to ask specific questions. One doctor picked up the phone and called me at work to ask, "Where did you see my article?" She was unaware it had been published on the internet.

Now that I was in control, I transferred my care to a well-known breast surgeon with Baptist Health Systems, much closer to my home. I read the notes from the Mount Sinai surgeon suggesting a "re-cut" but instead my new surgeon advised me to consider a "Total Axillary Node Dissection" (TAND) – the removal of all the lymph nodes – since my sentinel lymph node had been positive. This method assured that no stray nodes were harboring cancer cells, but it also came with some side effects like 1-in-3 chances of lymphedema (painful swelling of the arm). After my physician gave me the choice, I opted for the TAND because I wanted the most aggressive approach. I also met with an astute, professional oncologist, who agreed with me and ordered an aggressive,

dose-dense (meaning, every two weeks, rather than standard three) chemotherapy regimen. Since the triple negative cells were grade 3 (fast growing) I wanted the best effective proven therapy.

One week after my first chemo treatment I experienced a mild headache at work. My chemo class taught us to always take our temperature with any headache and I was shocked when the thermometer read 101.3. I ended up in the oncologist's office after hours and was quickly rushed off to the emergency room when my absolute neutrophil count (ANC) and white count were bottomed out. After my fever went even higher and blood cultures were taken, I was diagnosed with neutropenic fever and admitted to South Miami Hospital (the only one with beds available), where I began shaking uncontrollably with high fever and feeling generally miserable.

The timing was very bad. The following day, a new tropical depression intensified into Tropical Storm Katrina and headed westward toward Florida, strengthening into a hurricane only two hours before making landfall. The windows across the hall from my room in South Miami Hospital shattered and the power went out. My hospital bed was stuck in the upright position and my IV antibiotics stopped dripping. When I got home, we were still without power, but I realized how fortunate we were when I saw what Katrina was doing to the New Orleans area. I thought of other cancer patients who might be receiving treatment and what they were going through.

Ultimately, thirty-six radiation therapy visits decreased my immune system even lower. That's when I knew I had to do something.

ALONG CAME ALICE

Seven years out of breast cancer treatment, my immune system was still not close to normal. The oncologist did a bone marrow biopsy, which didn't show any abnormalities. As I began researching the immune system following chemo and radiation for breast cancer I was enticed by articles I read on boosting your immune system to assist in keeping the cancer in NED (No Evidence of Disease).

At the same time an interesting, energetic woman named Alice Billman visited the Bosom Buddies support group to discuss The Heroines Choir. She described the choir's positive mission of improving health by healing mind, body, and spirit through learning the art of choral singing and performance. Alice informed us that singing helps build up the immune system and causes new synaptic activities of the brain by learning to read and sing music, while memorizing lyrics. Singing also gives the lungs a workout, toning abdominal muscles and the diaphragm, stimulating circulation and making us breathe more deeply. It works like many forms of exercise, forcing us to take in more oxygen, improving aerobic capacity and experiencing a release of muscle tension as well.

Six years ago, I attended the first THC (The Heroines Choir) practice. I was looking for something beyond a support group and wanted to try to boost my immune system so that cancer would never come into my life again. I had asthma all my life and I was also hoping to improve my asthma and breathing, in addition to the chemical sensitivities brought on by chemo.

As I learned later, there was a benefit for our audience also; we could show the newly diagnosed breast cancer patients that there was "life after cancer." I was impressed by the energy and enthusiasm of the professional voice teacher and the founder/artistic director. Alice started the choir after losing a dear friend to this cruel disease.

Music is perhaps the oldest mind-body therapy, practiced long before Yoga, Tai Chi or Qigong. Looking back in history, before doing those exercises, people were singing. I immediately felt a sense of familiarity and comfort in the choir, bringing back warm childhood memories of singing in school and church with my musical family. After the first practice, I knew this was my new passion and mission: to help heal myself and assist breast cancer survivors become breast cancer *thrivers*!

All choirs must do vocal warm ups but because Alice owns "Kung Fu Connection," she appropriately integrated Qigong, the Chinese art of breathing, into our routine. These are profound but gentle movements that train the body, mind and spirit. They calm the mood in the room, so we can really concentrate on our practice time.

Just seven short months later, The Heroines Choir performed in front of big crowds of supporters and survivors at the Race for the Cure, downtown Miami. Every time we performed, I felt the tremendous endorphin rush of being on-stage, but also the excitement and pleasure of the audience, enjoying the songs as much

as we did. I saw something in their eyes beyond just emotion; we were showing them they can not only survive breast cancer, but learn new activities, thrive and have fun again.

If you have experienced cancer and/or chemo, you are probably wondering how we memorize the lyrics, melodies, and choreography. "Chemo brain" is a real side effect of some of the strong chemo drugs used for breast cancer, especially TNBR. Research reveals that singing employs all parts of the brain and helps with memory issues.

I learned from my own investigation that beginning a new venture at age 65, like singing in a choir, wasn't too old. Greg Cohen, of George Washington University, tracked a Senior Singers Choral in Arlington, VA and noted, "The chorale singers' average age was 80 – the youngest being 65 and the oldest 96. Preliminary data shows singers suffer less depression, make fewer doctor's visits a year, take fewer medications and had increased their other activities".

Now I felt like a youngster, just starting this adventure in my mid-60s! And it is true that I increased my other activities, like water aerobics three times per week, just because I was feeling better and experiencing less fatigue.

I watched my immune system gradually return to almost normal and anxiously awaited every CBC (Complete Blood Work) in the oncologist's office. Over my years with the choir, I continued researching articles on its psychological benefits, including immune response for cancer patients. A 2016 article by the Faculty of Medicine, Imperial College in London, demonstrated that singing in

a choir can not only reduce depression and anxiety but reduce levels of stress hormones and improve immune function. In South Wales, five choirs were studied by testing saliva and blood samples. In all five, singing was associated with reductions in negative effect and increases in positive effect, alongside significant increases in cytokines and all the "feel good" chemicals.

Looking toward my seventh decade and beyond, I started thinking about retiring. Participation in The Heroines Choir gave me not only a newfound confidence to keep working, but the increased ability to "read" music, match a note, and learn new lyrics. Each new learning experience included a variety of venues where we sang in front of small-to-huge audiences, ranging from outdoor cancer events to an NBA Heat game, where we were honored to sing the National Anthem.

Many of our audiences included survivors at various stages. We have received feedback from that not only did they enjoy the choir, they now felt if we could get on stage and sing and dance during or after our cancer experiences, they could too.

Our audiences find The Heroines Choir inspirational. We don't pretend to be professional singers; just ordinary women who have invested our time to learn to sing. We have worked with ladies who have had every stage of cancer, including the initial anger, denial, and uncertainty of which treatment path to follow.

We have newly diagnosed and women with stage IV (metastatic) cancer. When we sang at the Cancer Support Community in Miami, a woman approached me afterwards and expressed interest in joining us. I had a strong feeling that she was near the end of her journey, although she never shared it. Her enthusiasm was evident: she helped us write a song when our directress was leaving, performed with us, and played the guitar. Unfortunately, she passed away shortly after. We grieved together as a group and even though her family didn't have a service, we dedicated a performance to her at one of our large events. I feel that THC made a small but significant difference in her last months.

According to Patty Mills, Public Relations for Yankee Maid Chorus in "Music Notes," life-affirming benefits of singing include:

- Increased Poise, Self-esteem and Presentation Skills

- Strengthened Concentration and Memory
- Development of the Lungs
- Promotion of Superior Posture
- Broadened Expressive Communication
- Enriched Speech with a More Pleasant Quality
- Animated Body, Mind, and Spirit
- Ability of performer to Delve into Characterization/Acting
- Stimulation of Insight into Prose and Poetry and Piqued Interest in the Inner Meaning of Words
- Enhanced Ability to Appreciate the Art of Great Singers
- Therapeutic Emotional and Physical Effects

Although the choir is very much a support group, we never really discuss our ailments and treatments; instead we use the rehearsal time to challenge our chemo brains with new learning experiences that keep us sharp. Some members learn quickly and sing beautifully, while the rest of us increase our knowledge with every practice – even in the shower and the car. If we don't feel ready for an event, we do "extra practices" in my office after work.

We have also formed a "Broadway Buddies" group that has season tickets to the Arsht Center for Performing Arts for Saturday matinees. We make it a day-long outing by enjoying a nice lunch together. Whether for choir practice or social activities, we always have fun and laugh a lot. We are offered tickets to all the University of Miami Frost School of Music events and attend many university functions as a group, furthering our knowledge of music and our friendship.

There are no excuses in the choir. We have no audition. Everyone who wants to join us is welcomed. Each of us has had our own journey: we do our best as we all learn a new skill of singing together in harmony in an inharmonious world. As a registered nurse, it amazes me that when we sing, our hearts begin to beat in unison, synchronized through our breathing and our harmony.

May 15, 2018 marked my 13-year CANCERTHRIVERVERSARY!

That's my own word to express how I feel. I am not celebrating cancer; I am rejoicing that I am a Survivor/Thriver!

I have confronted my mortality and I found a new way of living, driven by a new skill, and a new-found appreciation of life, with a camaraderie unlike any I have ever witnesses in my 71 years!

The mission of the choir is to improve the health and quality of living for participants and their supporters, while inspiring audiences through the art of chorale singing. In six short years we have met that mission and beyond.

Music creates a special bond that goes beyond words and lyrics. The women in the choir become like a close family, creating a community of healing and of hope. We meet on Sunday afternoons in a light, roomy space with a wonderful view of the fountains and gardens in the new Miami Cancer Institute. Soon, we will move to a specially designed "Music Room" which the design committee intended for groups like us.

The uniform for The Heroines Choir is flashy – bright pink capes over black t-shirts emblazoned with the eye-catching Heroines logo, conveying *power* and *confidence*. The capes have been a big trendsetter for other groups; especially as a visual in Miami, where the breeze frequently blows.

As Linda Burrowes, founder of *Your Bosom Buddies* said "the women in the choir are truly heroines and it is so inspirational how they thrive after joining The Heroines Choir. The camaraderie with other survivors and the healing effect of the music they sing is truly remarkable!"

The magical healing powers of music and singing have impacted our professional and personal lives in ways none of us could have imagined. We continue to learn, grow, perform, and experience the power of singing to heal, while gaining strength, improved health and endless joy.

"Music gives a soul to the universe, wings to the mind, flight to the imagination and life to everything"

— Plato

References

1. Fancourt, Daisy, Williamson, Aaron, and Carvalho, Livian *Singing modulates mood, stress, cortisol, cytokine and neuropeptide activity in cancer patients* London UK, Tenovous Cancer Care, Gleider House
2. Moss, Hilary, Lynch, Julie and O'Donahue, Jessica *Exploring the perceived health benefits of singing in a choir; an international cross-sectional mixed-methods study,* Perspectives in Public Health, May 2018 Vol 138 No 3
3. Nagarsheth, Nimesh *Music and Cancer, A Prescription for Healing,* Jones and Bartlett 2010
4. Wikipedia, Hurricane Katrina 2005
5. CURE magazine: "Fuel to the Fire" Breast Cancer Special Issue, 2017
6. Kang J, Scholp A and Jiang J, Voice magazine, *A Review of the Physiological Effects and Mechanisms of Singing.*
7. Mills, Patty, *Vocalizing Promotes Well Being* "Music Notes" Fairfield/New Haven January 2000

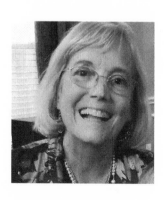

Marilyn Van Houten R.N., M.S., C.C.M. is a Registered Nurse with 50 years of extensive nursing, rehab, advocacy, and case management experience, and a 13-year, Triple Negative Breast Cancer "thriver." She founded her case management company, Rehab Case Management, where she has successfully helped to rehabilitate workers comp and catastrophic injury patients for the past 28 years.

Diagnosed with the most aggressive type of Breast Cancer in 2005, she found herself on a pathway to not only research the recently discovered TNBC phenotype, but also became the Assistant Director of The Heroines Choir, a group of cancer survivors and friends. She is passionate about improving health and healing mind, body and spirit through the art of chorale singing.

She received the *Case Manager of the Year Award* by the local CMSA chapter for her advocacy of breast cancer patients. Currently she is serving on the PFAC (Patient Family Advisory Council) of the Miami Cancer Institute (MCI) and has served on the committee to design the building, as well as chairing the Survivorship Committee.

As an R.N. with national Case Management certification and a "thriver/survivor" she is keenly aware of the importance of advocating, mentoring and guiding patients, who have faced breast cancer.

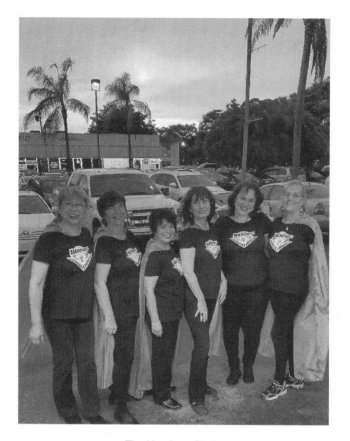

The Heroines Choir.

25

PEACE OF MIND PLANNING: THE LEGAL SIDE OF THINGS

JONATHAN DAVID, ESQUIRE

Why the need for planning?
(a/k/a "If you don't tell them, they won't know.)

You knew you were going to see it, and so here it is... the legal disclaimer! Despite the great info and guidance in this chapter, the author strongly recommends that you seek the counsel of a competent attorney specializing in estate planning to draft legal documents referred to in this chapter, and to understand your needs. For some convincing in this regard, see the sections entitled "Cautionary Tales" [or "War Stories" – haven't decided – JD].

Your planning for a future eventuality is all about *speaking now*, in anticipation of a time in the future when you may not be able to speak for yourself. Without wanting to sound too much like the author of a sci-fi novel, think of your planning documents as letters to the people of the future, to be read at a time when necessary.

With whom in this future time are you communicating? Anyone! Doctors, judges, family, friends... And what are you saying to them? Anything! (just about).

Telling people around you what you want them to do (or know) includes:

- Advising doctors what to do/not to do to you while you're undergoing treatment;
- Appointing a trusted person to manage your affairs in case you can't;
- Telling a judge whom you want to be in charge of your *estate*;
- Advising your family/estate executor whether you want to donate organs, the kind of funeral or memorial service you'd like to have (including disposition of your remains);
- Telling the judge whom you want to take care of your minor children (if the co-parent is not fulfilling that role) and whom you want to have your possessions;
- Passing the baton on obligations, maintenance of your home and/or business, and other projects, for as-smooth-as-possible continuation: What do your successors need to know? Have you planned for continuing payment of your home mortgage? Do you run a business?

Summary

There might be a lot more to take care of than you realize (a lot more of a mess than you think, that needs to be cleaned up after you). Creating adequate planning documents will minimize problems and uncertainty for those managing your affairs when you are unable to do so. Whether the intended objects of your planning documents are family members, friends, business associates, doctors, or a probate judge, making a clear record of what you want to be done will save a lot of wondering, guessing, bickering and problems.

Further along in this chapter, I'll explain what the *probate* process is, and define the words "probate", "guardianship," etc., but first, let me list and describe some common planning documents:

Planning Documents

It's helpful to be acquainted with the basic planning vehicles. Here are the most used documents, with a brief explanation of each:

Power of Attorney: This is a document in which you (the "principal," in legal nomenclature) designate a person who can act for you – in your place – to do various things, while you are alive. The person to whom you designate the authority to act for you is known as your "attorney-in-fact". This person doesn't have to be a lawyer. The word "attorney" in this phrase simply means someone authorized to speak and act on your behalf.

Common examples of possible uses for a power of attorney might be:

- My mother signs a power of attorney giving me the power to withdraw money from her bank account. In the event that she becomes incapacitated and her home bills need to get paid, I can do that for her;
- I know that I will be traveling out of the country on the day of closing on the sale of a house I own, so I sign a power of attorney specifically giving a friend of mine the authority to sell my house – to sign any deed, bill of sale, closing/settlement statement, etc., and deposit the money into my account.

So, if there are things you think might need to get done (without court intervention), and you know of a trusted relative or friend who might be able to take care of those things, a power of attorney is a vehicle that can accomplish that.

A *durable* power of attorney refers to a power of attorney that specifically has a clause declaring that it should stay in force even if the person who signed it becomes incapacitated – something like this: "[THE EFFECTIVENESS OF] THIS DURABLE POWER OF ATTORNEY IS NOT AFFECTED BY THE SUBSEQUENT INCA-

PACITY OF THE PRINCIPAL, EXCEPT AS PROVIDED BY APPLIC-ABLE LAW." This clause ensures that whoever is relying on the Power of Attorney knows that it remains effective even if the person who gave it is undergoing treatment in the hospital, unconscious, or unable to act for some other reason (other than death! See next section entitled "CAUTION").

CAUTION: A power of attorney loses its power upon the death of the person who gives it! For that reason, it can't be a substitute for a Law Will & Testament. It won't even allow the designated attorney-in-fact to withdraw money from a bank account after the death of the principal.

CAUTION #2: A power of attorney can be abused by the person to whom it is granted. Of course, it is illegal for the designated "attorney-in-fact" to use the power of attorney for his own benefit and/or to the detriment of the principal, but, sadly, it is not uncommon. Make sure that person you designate is trustworthy. Some people keep the power of attorney in a "safe" place at home, and tell the attorney-in-fact where it can be found in the event of the incapacity of the principal. As long as the attorney-in-fact has access to the principal's home when the time comes, this is a safe and effective approach.

Living Will

"Living Will" is the common name for an Advanced Healthcare Directive. It's a document that instructs doctors and health care providers about what you do and don't want done to you in the event that you become incapacitated and cannot give the instructions directly. Common examples are: requesting (or requesting that the doctors withhold) life-support measures such as feeding tubes and breathing tubes.

The form of the document can vary. Sometimes a Power of Attorney includes the designation of a "health care surrogate" – a person chosen to make medical decisions on the spot. If you know where you are most likely to be treated (the nearest hospital, or your

regular physician(s), for instance) it is best to have a form that particular hospital recognizes. The legal departments of some hospitals are
picky about the exact language that they require (possibly based
upon recent local law that has evolved), although any institution
should honor a validly executed power of attorney.

Last Will and Testament:

This is a document, *executed with the formalities that your state's law
prescribes* (the proper number of witnesses, etc.), to tell a judge what
to do with your property, and whom you want in charge of managing
the collection, maintenance and distribution of your assets. It can
also contain some instructions or statements of desire concerning
non-property matters, such as designating who should take care of
your minor children in a situation where the co-parent is not able to
do so. It is intended to be a document formally processed ("probat-
ed") by the court system. In the absence of a *last will & testament*, each
state has laws dictating which family members get what portion of
your assets (called "laws of intestacy"). Such a law might say, "spouse
gets half and children share the other half," or "if a person dies
having no spouse or children, then the estate is shared by decedent's
siblings."

Why you need a will:

- **For certainty:** Whenever a person dies without a will, one
  preliminary step is *making sure that there isn't* a will. That
  is, if a probate judge asks, "Are you sure that this person
  did not have a will?" the only way to be 100% sure is to rifle
  through all personal effects – shaking books, looking
  under mattresses – that kind of thing – until you can say
  for sure that "after diligent search, no known will could be
  found." When there is a signed, sealed and delivered
  document with "Last Will & Testament" on its face, the
  court has a clear starting place to begin its proceedings;

- **To designate the person or persons you wish to manage your affairs** and act as your executor. Family members could fight over who should be in charge of your estate/probate affairs;
- **Because law changes** from time to time, and if you rely on what you *think* the law governing intestacy is, it may not be the same at the time of your death. But it's best not to leave it to a law that could change with every sitting of your state's legislature.
- **Designation of a guardian for your minor child(ren):** Making sure that the decision of who should raise your kid(s) is not left up to a court hearing where two sides of the family (the in-laws!) sling mud to convince a judge that they are the better surrogate parents than those unbearable people on the other side of the courtroom;
- **To communicate any special desires:** for your pets, for your funeral, etc. In such cases, your statements of desire may not be practically legally enforceable, but you can let them be known. For example, you may communicate how you wish your funeral to be conducted, but by the time the matter gets to court, your funeral would probably have already been conducted. To the extent that pets are considered "possessions" ("chattel" in legalese), you can devise (or bequeath or convey) them in your will, but you can't necessarily make sure that the person who inherits them take care of them.

THE PROBATE PROCESS

What is *probate* and how is it handled?

We've all watched the classic scene in a movie: the family gathers around in the family lawyer's office and listens as the lawyer reads the loved one's will aloud. In real life this happens very rarely. Usually when the time comes, the decedent's will is quietly filed with the court, and a proceeding (known as "probate") is begun. The word "probate" is from the Latin *probatum*, which means "a thing proved" (referring to the will itself, which is proved up in court). The steps include:

1. Presenting papers to the court;
2. Establishing who is entitled to notifications of court goings-on;
3. Appointment of the most appropriate person to act as executor (also sometimes called the "personal representative") to manage the estate case. This executor has to report to the court with an inventory of the decedent's assets, and will be in charge of collecting or paying debts, gathering ("marshaling") the assets of the decedent, selling property, etc.
4. Determining who gets paid what;
5. Actually distributing the assets to the appropriate people.

Even though it may be notarized and look about as official as a document can get, a beneficiary can't simply go to a 3rd party and present the will to receive his inheritance. Ask any bank officer if he or she has ever had a person (heir) come into the bank with a relative's last will & testament, present it to the bank officer and demand the money they are entitled to under the will. The bank has to turn the heir away, declaring, "We can't just acknowledge this will as dispositive (the final word). We need a court order directing us to give you the money."

Exceptions: Not everything needs a judge's involvement to transfer ownership

All of the above having been said, there are lots of assets that pass "outside the estate" – without the need for probate.

Some things are not considered estate assets: some assets pass directly, either by operation of law or by private contract, to other people, upon the happening of certain contingencies. Some examples are:

- bank accounts that specifically designate a "pay on death" beneficiary or accounts which are held jointly with another person with rights of survivorship;
- life insurance policies that name a specific beneficiary, who, by contract, is paid the benefit directly (not through the court);
- real property (house or land) owned by spouses (sometimes, whether the deed says to or not), or real property held with title (deed) designating a survivor owner;
- "homestead" (usually the primary home of a person) and other property with very specific local laws about who inherits it automatically, and may even prevent a person from disposing of it through a will.

If a life insurance policy names no one as the beneficiary (or designates only the person whose life is insured as the beneficiary), the matter must go through probate. Since the payee beneficiary (the very person whose life was insured) is now gone, how can the insurance company send them a check for the life insurance proceeds? In this case, the life insurance benefit goes into a special estate account, and is dealt with as part of the total assets of the decedent. The court either follows instructions in the last will and testament or local laws of intestacy to determine who should get that life insurance money.

What's all the hullabaloo about TRUSTS?

It's true that the probate process (going through all court procedures) can take a long time, even years in many cases. It can also be costly in terms of attorney's fees. For this reason, people try to devise ways to avoid the probate process and the court system altogether. One of those methods is a trust.

A trust is a device (usually a written agreement) through which one person holds property for the benefit of another person, with a set of instructions for what to do with that property. For example, the title to your house could be transferred (signed over, or "deeded") over to a *trustee*. Even though the trustee's name is now on the deed to your house, it is understood and agreed, in this scenario, that the trustee is only holding the property for you. The instructions to the trustee may be along the lines of: "If something happens to me, sell the house and distribute the proceeds equally between my nieces and nephews." Since the title-holder to the property (the trustee) is alive and empowered to sell the house, it can be done without delay that a court proceeding can occasion.

Wow. That sounds great. Why doesn't everyone do a trust?

Yes, a trust can prevent certain delays posed by the court process. But here's the reality: everything is a double-edged sword. For the flexibility one gains by not going through probate, one loses the court oversight and the transparency that a court proceeding gives. Also, there can be snags, if one is not careful. If the trust agreement (the document itself) is lost, then the family could end up with a situation where a trustee is holding property but doesn't know what he is supposed to do with it. And the trust has to be *funded* – that is, the title to assets must be changed to name the trust/trustee as the new owner. Often enough, people pay an attorney to draft a trust, but then the person creating the trust forgets to transfer assets into it. And lastly, but not least: if your trustee turns out to be untrustworthy, you may end up in court after all, when it is too late to prevent some loss.

GUARDIANSHIP: The law's formalities for taking care of those who can't take care of themselves.

If you were to find yourself unable to manage your affairs and you didn't have a designated attorney-in-fact (through a power of attorney, described above), nor a health care surrogate to make decisions for you, you could find yourself in a position where the court must appoint a *guardian* to manage your personal (physical) affairs and finances. Your guardian acts kind of like a parent, making sure you have what you need, and in some ways stands in your shoes, since your guardian (with court approval) can transact business and make decisions that you would if you could.

The legal process for accomplishing the appointment of a guardian is, very generally stated, the filing of the appropriate papers with the court, and a hearing in court (after notifications to all interested persons) where it is determined whether or not the prospective *ward* (the person to be protected or cared for) needs a guardian. If it is determined that a guardian is needed, the court will try to choose the most appropriate person or professional caregiving company to fill that role. A guardianship may be very limited in scope, or the court may declare that a person is completely in need of care (lacks the capacity to act for herself in any degree), in the areas of personal physical care and/or management of financial matters. In those cases where a guardian is appointed, the court requires the guardian to file periodic reports to ensure that the ward is being taken care of, and that any powers given to the guardian (including financial management powers) are not being abused.

Some jurisdictions have a procedure established for declaring a "pre-need guardian." This is accomplished through a written document which clarifies your preference for a guardian to manage your affairs if you should become incapacitated (we used to say "incompetent" but that word is frowned upon now). It is a formal statement (observe any legal formalities required!) and is filed with the Clerk of Court in your county of residence. You can then have some peace of mind knowing that if you become incapacitated, someone you know and trust will take care of you.

MAKING AN INVENTORY

In this section, I list some of the main things you may want to consider, just as a starting point for formal planning, and maybe for your attorney to use to help in drafting any documents. The idea is to evaluate what you own, and to ask yourself what you envision doing with it. Once you have completed this task of creating a list, it important to let someone trusted know about it! Your family and friends could overlook something if they are unaware of its existence.

Assets: All physical (personal property and real estate) and intangible (stocks, accounts, insurance) things you own.

- Real estate: Making sure you don't lose it for failure to make the mortgage payments, and deciding what you want to do with it
- Life insurance: Making sure it does not lapse; Designating the most appropriate beneficiary(ies).
- Business Interests: Making a plan for operation in your absence or succession.
- Jewelry
- Intellectual Property?

What to do with each item:

- Sell?
- Give away while living (*inter vivos* transfer?
- Devise? (that is, provide for in will?)
- Donate organs?

Debts

Passing on the responsibility for making mortgage payments (or having family member re-finance). It's a pity when a house goes into foreclosure because no one steps up to take care of that.

Taxes

Don't forfeit your home for failure to pay real estate taxes.

IRS? Information that would be needed for a final tax return.

Funeral/Burial Plans:

Preferred funeral home?

Preferred method of disposition?

Who's paying? When?

Notification: Who should be notified about your death (many times, the loved one's family doesn't know the names of old friends)?

Charity donations in lieu of flowers?

What information should be included in the obituary?

War stories from a practitioner:

In my years of practicing law, I've come across some doozies – stories I keep in my mental files and re-tell to make valid points. Here are a few of the general narratives to give you a sense of some potential pitfalls:

Lost Estate Documents

If no one around you can find your estate-planning documents, then they do no good! There are cases where the family finds a will in a hiding place at a time when it is too late – when the probate case is already long over and done with. There are also cases, as briefly alluded to above, where some property/asset is put into the name of a trust, but then later no one can find the Trust Agreement setting out what was to be done with the trust's property.

Some people assume that the attorney who drafts the estate documents will keep an original or copy of the papers – somehow committing to act as a depository -- but this is not necessarily the case. And anything can happen even to a lawyer's papers: destruction in a fire, files getting moldy in a storage facility, etc. Therefore, you will want to find a safe place for your documents, or make/keep multiple originals to share with trusted family members.

If you have a safe deposit box, that is a good place for your important documents, but don't forget to *tell someone* close to you that the safe deposit box exists, and at what bank branch. In one of my probate cases, long after it was determined that the last will could not be found, a piece of mail arrived from a bank – an invoice for annual renewal of a safe deposit box that the next of kin knew nothing about. A court order authorizing the opening of the safe deposit box in front of witnesses (to take an inventory of the contents) yielded the discovery that there was, in fact a will in the box. Luckily it was not too late in that case.

Do-it-yourself Last Will & Testament

One of my favorites is the occasional phone call from someone saying, "I've just written and signed a will. Can you look at it and tell me if it's OK?" Do I need to tell you that *after* signing is not the time to be getting an attorney's opinion about a document that has legal effect?! Although there is nothing necessarily invalid about a will that you have drafted on your own, there are enough lawyers around, and it is easy enough to avoid a lamentable outcome.

Minors Getting Their Hands on Big Money at a Young Age

In my practice, I have been involved in a guardianship cases in which the minor child receives a substantial sum, whether through life insurance from a parent, settlement of a personal injury lawsuit, or inheritance. In such cases, the court monitors and protects the minor's money, keeping it in a court-restricted account, and requiring annual reporting to the court that the money is still there, safe and sound. *But these guardianship cases terminate when the minor reaches age*

18, and the court, by law, has to turn the money over to the young minor-turned-adult, who can then do with it whatever he or she pleases.

In all too many of these instances, an 18 year-old comes into an amount of money he or she really doesn't know how to manage. The young adult often blows through the money frivolously in short order – on expensive cars (sometimes later wrecking them, without insurance in place), loans to friends, bad investments, or living an unsustainable lifestyle .

To prevent something like that from happening to, say, the life insurance benefit that may be paid to your minor beneficiary or beneficiaries, a *trust* is a useful tool. Instead of naming a minor beneficiary on your life insurance policy, you name **the trust** as the beneficiary. You can then have a trust agreement which instructs your trustee to make payments to your beneficiaries over time, with any schedule you can envision and establish, such as:

Trustee shall pay to Beneficiary:

- $3,000 per month while Beneficiary is in college
- $10,000 upon graduation from college
- $35,000 upon reaching age 23
- $50,000 upon Beneficiary reaching age28
- The balance of any remaining funds upon Beneficiary reaching a certain age

The trust could also have discretionary terms (things left up to the trustee) and could provide for payments to third parties for health and education of the beneficiary.

War Story: Trusting a Family Member to Distribute Funds

Sometimes a client will tell me that he or she intends to leave a life insurance policy to one child, and *that* child will share (divide and distribute) it amongst his or her siblings. This works fine if the child really *does* it (setting aside any possible tax consequences to the child who receives the funds). But how can you know if it will really be done? I have had cases where family members come to me claiming that the sibling who was supposed to share what he or she was given is not doing so. In such cases, it is an uphill battle to sue the recalcitrant sibling for refusal to share.

CONCLUSION: Gazing Into the Future

Wouldn't it be great if we all had a crystal ball? One that could accurately predict the future and tells us in specific terms exactly what's going to happen, what we need to worry about, and what will resolve itself?

Unfortunately, none of us has an all-knowing crystal ball; therefore, we must plan ahead. Regardless of the apparent urgency of the situation, creating a plan now is the way to ensure that as much of your affairs and wishes as possible become effectuated, and that the complications and uncertainty are minimized.

∾

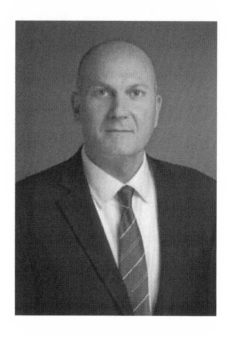

Jonathan Noble David is a Miami-based attorney and mediator specializing in estate planning and inheritance matters. A native of Coral Gables and a graduate of Duke University (bachelors) and University of Miami School of Law, Mr. David has been practicing for over 20 years, and prides himself on being conscientious, practical, and possessing the ability to convey concepts to his clients without the using more legalese than necessary, and focusing on a more human approach to legal questions. He can be reached at jdavd@southmiamilegal.com. His law firm's web address is www.southmiamilegal.com

26

RESOURCES

Living Beyond Breast Cancer
10 East Atthes Avenue, Suite 204
Ardmore, PA 19003
Phone - 610-645-4567
FAX - 610-645-4573
http://www.lbbc.org

Living Beyond Breast Cancer, founded in 1991, is a national nonprofit organization dedicated to empowering all women affected by breast cancer to live as long as possible with the best quality of life. Programs and services include:

- Conferences;
- Teleconferences;
- Toll-free Survivor's Helpline (1-888-753-5222);
- Website lbbc.org;
- Free quarterly newsletters;
- Publications for African-American and Latina women;
- Recordings;

- Networking programs;
- Healthcare-provider trainings;
- and the Paula A Seidman Library and Resource Center.

1. The Susan G. Komen Breast Cancer Organization
2. http://www.komen.org
3. Young Survival Coalition (YSC)
4. Phone 646-257-3000 - toll free - 1-800-972-1011
5. LympheDIVAS, founded by RachelTroxell http://www.lymphedivas.com
6. FORCE (Facing Our Risk Of Cancer Empowered)
7. http://www.facingourrisk.org/index.php
8. Positively Pat - founder Patricia San Pedro www.postivelypat.com
9. Facebook Link of Hope Sistas Support Group www.facebook.com **Note:** This is a private group; use the search feature on Facebook to look it up and request to join.
10. American Cancer Society http://www.cancer.org
11. Beatriz Amendola, M.D. Innovative Cancer Institute http://www.innovativecancer.com/oncologist/beatriz-e-amendola-md-pa

EPILOGUE

Dear Life,

   As I get closer to birthday number 64, where many contemplate retirement and others do not have the privilege to see, I think about getting older and where my life is heading. I never thought I would get to this age. I remember the day I turned 13 thinking how cool it was to become a teenager. That was a fun time in life, when everyone played together and there were no cell phones or computers. Over the years, I have experienced a miscarriage and a hysterectomy, and losing both breasts, my father, and my brother to cancer. Yet I realize I still have much to be grateful for, including the amazing people in my life. I thank God and all of you who have supported my work as an advocate and been there for me whenever I had meltdowns. I am forever grateful. I welcome my next birthday on July 6 and look forward to celebrating it with the close friends I consider family.

In love and gratitude,
Cindy